# Praise for
## America's Most Dangerous Jobs

"*America's Most Dangerous Jobs* focuses on the men and women who do our country's essential work—jobs that put their lives and health in jeopardy. Dr. Robert Larsen provides a straight-up look at workers who have been injured—often through no fault of their own—while doing what they have to do. These narratives opened my eyes to the risks that construction crews, farmers, emergency responders, highway maintenance crews, roofers, landscapers, and workers in many other professions face daily.

In his psychiatric practice, Dr. Larsen sat with workers injured on the job in accidents that changed their lives forever. The way the workers handle these traumatic challenges speaks to the unbearable weight of suffering in some cases and to the gift of resilience in others. Each unique story is told with both truth and compassion."

— Anne Hillerman, author of the best-selling Leaphorn, Chee, and Manuelito mysteries; Executive producer *Dark Winds*

"Overall, a definite winner. You have captured some of the toughest jobs and what our patients have to sacrifice every time they clock in. It is truly amazing that we are all hanging on by a thread. If you get through life unscathed, or relatively unharmed, it is a true blessing and miracle."

— Michael Post, M.D., Medical Director, RehabOne Medical Group; Past President, California Society of Industrial Medicine & Surgery

"In his new book, *America's Most Dangerous Jobs,* Dr. Bob Larsen opens your eyes to the many professions working around you every day and the risks those workers take carrying out their duties. Dr. Larsen describes cases where workers from 25 different professions are injured on the job. In vignettes, he discusses the risks connected to specific professions, case examples where an injury occurred, and often includes information on how the person responded to the injury. This fascinating book will certainly change the way you look at the people performing necessary but dangerous jobs."

— Joel Fay, Ph.D., Founding Member, First Responders Support Network; Lead Clinician, West Coast Post-Trauma Retreat

"Dr. 'Bob,' as his colleagues fondly call him, reminds us of how tenuous our health can be and how a single incident can plunge us into the abyss of despair, dysfunction, and chronic pain. His advocacy for injured workers, over many decades, is well known. He advises us to 'Count your blessings rather than focus on how life could be better' and 'Don't live in fear of injury and insult.' This book is a must-read!"

— Steven D. Feinberg, M.D., M.P.H., M.S., Adjunct Clinical Professor, Stanford University, School of Medicine

"In a digital age where many information-economy employees work remotely, it is easy to forget how dangerous many of the jobs are that keep our society running. Attorneys and doctors in the workers' comp system see many of these workers whose lives are upended by injury events on their jobs. Bob Larsen's book is a compelling look at workers injured on some of the most dangerous jobs. With compassion and insight, he tells stories of how these events shaped their lives and the lives of their families."

— Julius Young, Esq., Senior Partner, Boxer & Gerson, LLP

# Dedication

This book, like its predecessor, *Wounded Workers*, is dedicated to all workers who produce goods, provide services, and administer systems in America while risking their lives, physical health, and emotional well-being.

# Privacy Statement

I have made a sincere effort to preserve the privacy of those whose tales are told. What follows in these nonfiction narratives are accurate depictions of sagas told to me by folks who fell upon misfortune while doing their jobs. This usually occurred through no fault of the worker. There is no basis for blame or shame.

As in *Wounded Workers,* the identities of workers who are the subjects of *America's Most Dangerous Jobs* have been protected. Names were changed. Employers' names were often altered. Time frames are not usually specified. Those modifications preserve confidentiality.

Essential aspects of the injury events have been preserved. This includes how the injury took place, what treatment was rendered, the approximate age of the worker, and the job title or nature of the worker's duties.

— Dr. Bob Larsen

# AMERICA'S MOST
# DANGEROUS JOBS

# AMERICA'S MOST DANGEROUS JOBS

More Tales from a Working Man's Shrink

## DR. BOB LARSEN

Working Man's Press

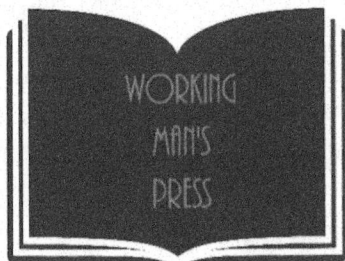

Working Man's Press

*America's Most Dangerous Jobs: More Tales from a Working Man's Shrink*
© 2025 by Robert C. Larsen

Book Design: Jordan Jones
Cover Design: Graphic Sky Printing

Working Man's Press
P. O. Box 31193
Santa Fe, NM 87594
https://workingmansshrink.com/
https://www.facebook.com/workingmansshrink

ISBN:   978-1-7348175-4-6 (hardcover)
        978-1-7348175-5-3 (paperback)
        978-1-7348175-6-0 (e-book)

**Disclaimer:** This book is not designed to and does not provide medical advice, diagnostic assessment, treatment or other clinical services. *America's Most Dangerous Jobs*, its website linkages, the author Robert C. Larsen, and the publisher Working Man's Press provide information for reading and educational purposes only. The information provided is not a substitute for medical or psychiatric care, and you should not use it in place of consultation or advice from your physician or health care providers. Dr. Larsen and Working Man's Press are not responsible for any clinical advice, diagnosis, treatment, products, or services you obtained by reading this book. Neither the Food and Drug Administration nor any other government agency has evaluated statements made in this book.

# Contents

# Foreword by Dr. David Baron

I first met Robert Larsen, Dr. Bob, over forty years ago when we were both Laughlin Fellows of the American College of Psychiatrists. Over the past four decades we have maintained our friendship. In addition to his expertise as a dedicated occupational psychiatrist, Dr. Bob is a passionate advocate for his patients and his beloved San Francisco Giants. He has shared his knowledge and passion in two books, *Wounded Workers* and his most recent work, *America's Most Dangerous Jobs.*

Dr. Bob sent me an advance copy of his new book, for comment. Ironically, I was in the process of reviewing the text when it was destroyed while in my home office, by the Eaton Fire. Since that devastating January 7th blaze, I have had the opportunity to interact with many of the first responders involved. Those heroes put their lives at risk to fight the fire while saving others and property when they could. My interactions with those professionals would have fit nicely in Chapter Seventeen of this text.

This nonfiction narrative provides a series of short clinical vignettes highlighting different aspects of the potential perils of the twenty-five most dangerous jobs in America. The reader is given an insider view and clinical perspective not available elsewhere. In typical Dr. Bob fashion, a genuine passion and concern for these workers comes out loud and clear.

I am very pleased to report the public concern and gratitude for all first responders involved in fighting the historic Southern California fires, Palisades, Eaton and Hughes, was extensive, and much appreciated by the firefighters on the front lines. It made a palpable difference to them and hopefully will have a carry-over effect moving forward.

This public response is not always the case in other dangerous professions, as the text points out. Enjoy the read and be on the lookout for Dr. Bob's next enlightening work on this important topic.

— David Baron, M.D.
   Professor of Psychiatry, Western University of Health Sciences
   Adjunct Clinical Professor of Psychiatry, Stanford University
   Professor, Public Health Research, Claremont University

# Introduction

This book continues the tales of our country's workforce that I began in *Wounded Workers: Tales of a Working Man's Shrink.* It tells the stories of workers subjected to stress, challenges and, at times, opportunities.

*America's Most Dangerous Jobs* tells tales of occupations found to have the highest fatality and serious injury rates in the U.S. I have described real cases referred over the years to my psychiatric practice that exemplify the risks workers in these job categories are subjected to.

The Bureau of Labor Statistics (BLS) periodically publishes a census of fatal occupational injuries.[1] Advisor Smith, which provides research and information on business insurance, uses the BLS data to identify the most dangerous job categories across the country.[2] The fatality rates based upon Advisor Smith's methodology were published in *Industrial Hygiene News*.[3] Other organizations, such as CNBC, rely upon the BLS for reporting on common workplace deaths.[4] I used these sources of information to compile the list of dangerous jobs that I cross-referenced with cases from my psychiatric practice. As there is no absolute consensus, there is no agreed upon order of "the most dangerous" as this concept incorporates fatality rates and the incidence of serious injuries.

An observant reader may become concerned that more cases of men than of women are told in this nonfiction narrative. It turns out that men are at increased risk for serious injury and death compared to their female co-workers. In 2022, 5,486 employees died because of work-related activities. Of these deaths, 445 were women and 5,041 were men. Roadway incidents were the number one cause of fatal accidents for both genders. However, women were twice as likely as their male co-workers to die from homicide when working.[5]

One measure of the severity of workplace injuries is the need for emergency medical services. According to the BLS and the Centers for Disease Control and Prevention, men account for two-thirds of E.R. visits for industrial injuries. A question to consider is whether men have more serious injuries or is there some bias in triaging men rather than women with similar injuries for emergency evaluation. Most of the serious injuries whose tales follow in this book are of men. That said, the challenges that women face when injured bring forth anxiety, moodiness, and uncertainty, as is the case for their male counterparts, when hurt for doing their jobs.

While I have conducted forensic psychological autopsies where a postmortem analysis is made of the facts related to an individual's cause of death, the cases in this book, except for one in Chapter 14, are of persons who survived though they were left with lingering traumatic repercussions. Post-traumatic stress disorder (PTSD) is a common condition seen in employees involved in critical incidents. Cops in gunfights, firefighters rescuing victims from fires, truck drivers in serious crashes, and teachers safeguarding pupils during mass shootings are examples of people whose lives are changed by workplace events.

As a physician, my goal is to be an advocate for workers exposed to life-changing and perhaps life-threatening stress and trauma. I take pleasure in assisting trauma victims to become survivors with a future. Like many reading this book, my life and way of doing business was altered by the COVID-19 pandemic. Many appointments for traumatized employees, which had been scheduled for weeks or months in our office, had to be postponed. In-person consultation was replaced with Zoom-interviews. Depositions on litigated cases took place at a distance. With the publication of *Wounded Workers*, I expected to give presentations to groups of doctors, attorneys, university audiences, and the public. This did happen, but in a manner I had not envisioned. I found myself appearing via software technology to audiences that included the School of Public Health at Johns Hopkins, the California Lawyers Association, the Santa Fe Public Library, and other organizations interested in these sagas.

My presentations are designed to be both informative and entertaining. Across all audiences, I try to convey three principles for conducting ourselves in various lines of work.

1. **Do no harm.** Don't make things worse for those who come to you.
2. **Walk in your neighbor's, client's, or patient's moccasins for a day.** Get to know someone before you try to change that person's life.

5

3. **Selectively advocate.** Not all interviewees need or deserve advocacy.

In my experience, it is often those who have experienced the most severe abuse or trauma who are neglected. They are the forgotten ones. We don't want to be reminded of our own vulnerability by being exposed in detail to what malice they were subjected to while just doing a job. Some of these tales are heartbreaking, at least at first. Others will give you hope. The tales are told to honor America's workers who may not appreciate the danger of the job functions they perform.

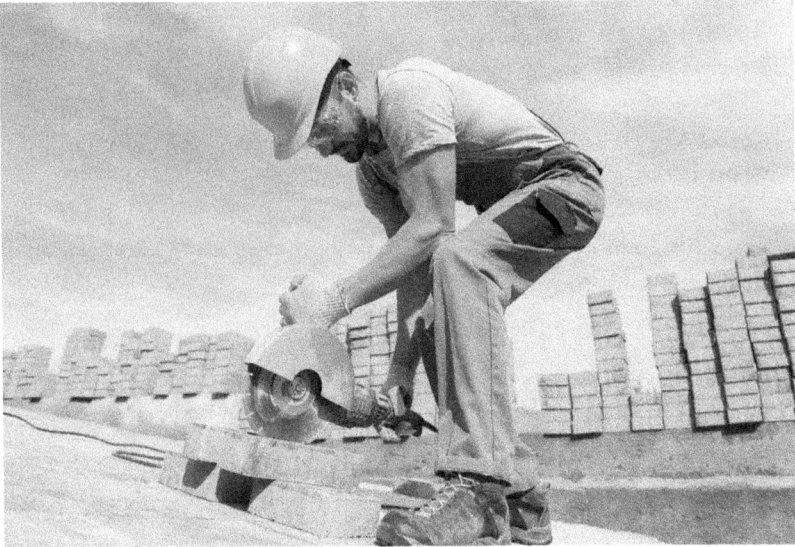

# 1    Construction Workers: At Risk When Building Things

## Construction Work is Risky Work

Working on a construction crew is inherently hazardous. The labor is strenuous. The machinery is powerful. The conditions can change. Notable hazards include working at heights, working in dusty conditions, using vibrating tools, and noise exposure.[1]

Construction workers are often exposed to a sensory overload of visual, auditory, olfactory, tactile, and other forms of input. Hot or cold environments can be the setting for a cacophony of sounds emitted by hammers pounding and power tools buzzing. Long workdays, work-related stressors, and disturbed sleep predispose these employees to depression and anxiety. Suicide is especially high among construction workers who typically do not make use of mental health services. The construction industry has the highest suicide rate of all professions.[2]

## The Case of Ali Kahn: Just One Misstep

Ali Kahn immigrated from the Middle East to California while in his early thirties. In his early years, he lived in a refugee camp with his parents and a dozen siblings. His father later operated a small retail shop. Ali was raised in the Muslim faith. He came to America for a better life and was pleased that he had relatives living in the Bay Area, where he came to live and work. He met his future wife, who was ten years his junior, through their mutual families. He had been a construction worker for two decades when he was injured.

For some years, Ali had worked for Like New Renovations, a construction company that improved distressed residential properties. On his first day working on a three-story home, Ali was pulling on a sheet of plywood on the structure's exterior, while standing on scaffolding a couple of stories above ground level. He lost his balance and fell to the concrete surface below. He lost his hardhat in the fall and struck his head, face, and neck on the hard surface where he landed.

Ali was taken to a major trauma center where he was hospitalized with a mild traumatic brain injury (TBI), a ruptured blood vessel inside his brain, a fractured left scapula, a cervical sprain, as well as multiple lacerations and contusions on the left side of his body and face. Awakening in the hospital, Ali was glad to be alive. As days went by, his post-traumatic headaches and bodily aches let him know he was in for a long struggle to regain what health he might.

8

We met more than two years after his fall. By then, Ali had not returned to the workforce. He was receiving a modest amount of disability benefits. He was living with other family members while his wife had gone to live with her parents. Ali was taking several analgesics, anti-inflammatory drugs, muscle relaxants, and other medications to deal with his headaches, chronic pain, and muscle spasms. He described having episodes of intense neck and low back pain that interfered with his ability to walk at times. He had avoided surgery, yet he no longer saw himself as having a future.

Not surprisingly, Ali's psychological test results were consistent with features of depression, anxiety, and somatic preoccupation. During our interview, he became openly tearful when asked to describe himself. While sobbing, he muttered, "I am broken."

I recommended a trial of an antidepressant to address his moodiness, disturbed sleep, and chronic pain. I encouraged him to make use of counseling for the very real concerns he had about his health, his work restrictions, and his personal life, as his estranged wife had filed for divorce. His legal claims would be resolved, but that would take time. It wasn't clear that Ali could be retrained for alternative employment because his physical impairment would not allow him to resume construction duties. He was likely to end up receiving Social Security Disability benefits.

The case of this construction worker makes clear how tenuous an employed person's existence can be. One day he or she has an accident at work and life changes. It's not surprising that Ali became depressed after he incurred his industrial injuries. He also was worried about heights, as he had never been before. This man struggled with self-blame, feelings of hopelessness, and suicidal thoughts.

*My great-grandfather died while working on a public works project in Chicago. He had yet to establish citizenship in the U.S. by the time of his death. His wife and children were deported back to Italy. Life is not always fair. Ali Kahn's family could understand that a worker's home life can suffer.*

## The Case of James Hill: Self-Described as Useless

For more than two decades, installing and maintaining power lines had been how James Hill spent his time working for a major public utility company. He had moved around to locations in central and northern California as required by his employer to work on major projects bringing in or updating high-voltage electrical lines. James got a sense of satisfaction at bringing progress to the communities his company served.

It was on a January morning when James was working on cutting the power to a line outside of Sacramento. He was electrocuted while using a power lift to access the line. One end of the live line had not been properly grounded. He reported, "I took 33,000 volts and survived." The worker was taken to a local trauma center. It was during that hospital stay that his cardiac rhythm had to be restored. Upon returning to the worksite within days, James was criticized by the on-site supervisor. "Look what you've done to my safety record!" His supervisor expressed no concern about James' health.

Having been electrocuted, James was referred for an evaluation of his injuries and any need for future care. The consulting physician recommended that James be assigned elsewhere with a different supervisor and in a location where he wouldn't worry about basic safety measures. Things went smoothly for about a year. James had worked on a project for more than two weeks without a day off when he experienced what he thought was a bad case of indigestion. He made an appointment with his pri-

10

mary care physician for the next day. His doctor diagnosed an acute myocardial infarction or heart attack. Arrangements were made for James to undergo coronary bypass surgery at a local hospital that day.

For a few months following his surgery, James took it easy at home. When he returned to his crew, he was assigned to light duty with his checking and organizing materials at the jobsite. He was allowed to continue with those tasks for several months. He again experienced what he then recognized as chest pain when engaging in more strenuous tasks one day at a construction site. At a follow-up visit with his cardiologist, James failed a cardiac stress test. He was no longer considered fit for duty. "They could have let me try to keep my job," he told me. The process began for this man to retire early due to disability. James stated, "I'm useless."

By the time I met James, he had been away from his work duties for about a year. He was convinced the electrocution event was what resulted in his heart attack and associated cardiovascular problems. It turned out that there was a strong family history of cardiac disease, his father having undergone bypass surgery. That parent had worked for the same utility company from which his son was now retiring. His health was being maintained with prescription medication for high blood pressure, elevated cholesterol levels, gout, osteoporosis, insomnia, depression, and combat-related PTSD. As a young man, he had been a member of the Army's 101st Airborne Division involved in horrific combat missions during the Vietnam War.

My psychiatric report could not find that James' emotional problems were primarily brought on by work because the cardiologists made a strong case for nonindustrial causes for his now chronic, and disabling, medical conditions. He was advised to pursue benefits for his service-connected exposure through the Veterans' Administration, given the obvious source of his post-traumatic memories, intrusive thoughts, and disturbing dreams. Ultimately, James' tale is common in our society where many employees are productive until they are physically worn out. Who wouldn't be dejected?

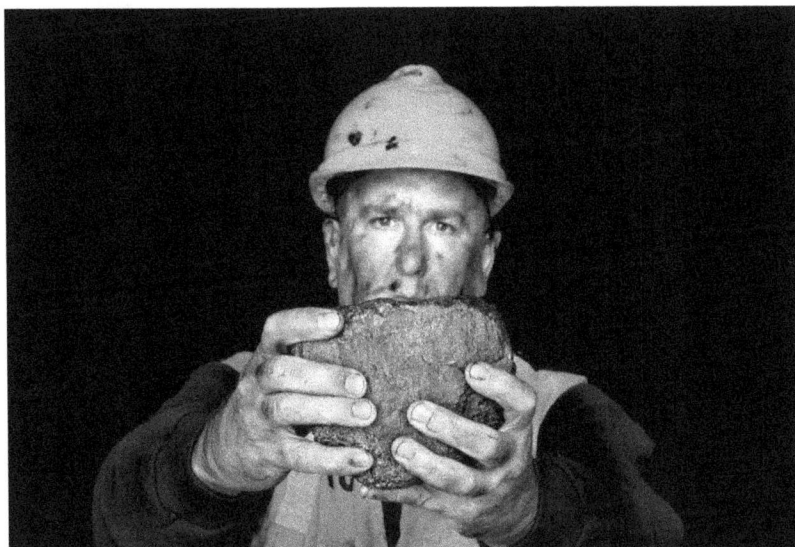

# 2   Mining Machine Operators: Dangerous Digging

## Risky Business

How much would you want to be paid to work underground? For many of us, the thought of working at heights is scary. Most folks would find work in a correctional facility, such as a state prison or county jail, to be unnerving, even for a day. For me, working as a roofer for one day was enough to cause me to quit before I got hurt. (See Chapter 22.) In this chapter, we consider the risks inherent in the jobs of miners and others who are employed below the surface of the earth.

There are all sorts of risks associated with operating heavy equipment. Machinery can malfunction. Operator error can be unforgiving. Conditions can change, bringing about unexpected accidents. When working below grade level, cave-ins are an ever-present danger. The thought of being buried alive would keep most people from working in mines. The states with the most active mines are Nevada, Arizona, and Wyoming.[1] U.S. mines extract heavy metals such as copper and zinc, precious metals like silver and gold, and minerals that include sulfur, and gravel.[2]

The vignettes that form the material for this book come from actual cases of workers referred to The Center for Occupational Psychiatry located in the San Francisco Bay Area. Miners and mining machine operators assume high-risk duties as do other mine workers. In this chapter, we examine the case of a laborer who was buried below grade and crushed when the walls of a deep trench collapsed onto him. There is also the case of a worker whose injuries were largely due to employer indifference and negligence with regard to safety measures.

## The Case of Jose Diaz: Trench Digging

Jose Diaz was born and raised in a rural part of Mexico. Most of his family were farm workers. One of six children, Jose had no formal education. He began working in the fields at an early age. Jose was a teenager when he came to live with his cousins in California's Central Valley. There, he picked fruit and vegetables, returning to Mexico in the off-season. As a young adult, Jose started working in construction. He picked up skills through on-the-job experiences over several years. He was hired by a pipeline company based in Fresno. The company was involved in installing pipes at construction projects and with large commercial farm irrigation.

Jose was working in a trench ten to twelve feet below ground level on the site of a residential project where his company was tasked with removing old pipes and replacing them with all new water and drainage lines. He was using a shovel and a pickax to remove the remaining dirt from around an old rotting drainage pipe when the sides of the trench gave way. The crew acted quickly using a backhoe and hand tools to extract Jose from the cave-in. He was rushed to a hospital where he remained unconscious for two days.

The laborer's hospital-based treatment required a surgical procedure to repair a fractured pelvis. A neurologist diagnosed a concussion and instituted treatment with an anticonvulsant, gabapentin, for post-traumatic headaches. He was told by the physician in charge of his care that he was lucky that his chest had not been crushed by the weight of the debris that surrounded him. Prior to discharge from the hospital, additional surgery was performed to address an inguinal hernia. A lengthy period followed the hospitalization. Jose's treatment was overseen by a physical medicine expert who prescribed physical therapy, chiropractic care, and prescription drugs that included narcotic analgesics, anti-inflammatory medication, muscle relaxants, a sedative, and trials of antidepressants. Jose was left with chronic pelvic, testicular, low back, and left leg pain.

Jose received temporary disability benefits from his employer's workers' compensation insurer. A co-worker had referred him to an attorney who represented him in a separate civil lawsuit. After a couple of years had passed, this injured worker still had significant limitations affecting his ability to walk more than a hundred feet without resting or to lift more than ten pounds. Jose, at the age of fifty, had been married to his wife for twenty years. His forty-year-old spouse is a seasonal employee of a local packing shed. The couple has three teenage children who are

U.S. citizens and help with household chores while still in high school.

Jose still has periodic traumatic dreams and found himself reminded of the cave-in when watching news coverage of an earthquake in Mexico. He has applied for Social Security Disability benefits, as the consensus of opinions is that combined physical and mental restrictions, along with his minimal amount of formal education, prevent this man from being a viable candidate for retraining and workforce re-entry.

The case of Jose Diaz is a reminder that, for some employees, a single injurious event can alter their life forever.

## The Case of Mike Barreto: Stuck Below Ground

Mike Barreto grew up in a Central California farming community where both of his parents were school bus drivers. He was the youngest of four kids in a working-class family of Portuguese origin. He understood the family surname came from the term "hatmaker" in his family's homeland. He wasn't aware of any family members who were involved in haberdashery. When seen in our offices, Mike was a somewhat portly fellow who was casually attired, wore a baseball cap on his shaved head, and used a cane to get around. He came across as a bit older than his stated age of forty-five.

It was Mike's last job that left him with a variety of musculoskeletal symptoms and complaints. He'd been injured before and was used to heavy labor activities, but his time with Jackson Industries had left him beat up and broken, in body and spirit. He took the job after being laid off from his duties on a ranch where he tended to flocks of sheep and goats, which he enjoyed. He knew that the job at Jackson involved tunneling and excavation beneath the ground level of the company's many garages and equipment sheds. These trenches or pits were used to service

16

trucks, tractors, and farm equipment such as harvesters. Jackson provided maintenance and repairs of farm vehicles and machinery. Mike was familiar with using backhoes from his days in the U.S. Army where he was assigned to an engineering unit.

Not long into his employment, Mike was asked to clean out waste from a service trench. There was more oil and discarded motor parts than he had expected. When he complained to the lead mechanic, he was told that his salary was adequate compensation for his getting "a bit dirty." Mike threatened to quit, but the general manager talked him out of doing so. In retrospect, the worker wished he trusted his assessment of a dangerous and poorly maintained worksite.

We met three years after Mike was in a service trench where he found a nest of Black Widow spiders. Taking a step back, his weight was too great for a wood plank floor that covered a 10-foot-deep pit that contained improperly stored petrochemicals that had been left on-site. With no co-workers in the area, Mike struggled to free himself from the quagmire where he came to rest, standing in sludge up to his arm pits. Luckily, there was an old wooden ladder that he commandeered for his escape. He was not merely filthy but bruised and lacerated from minor wounds on his face, hands, and arms. Taken to a local E.R., he made quite a sight before he was decontaminated in the process of that initial clinical encounter.

Over the year that followed his "pitfall," as Mike called the injury event, consultations were provided by orthopedic, internal medicine, chiropractic, occupational medicine, neurologic, and psychological experts. The consensus was that the worker had developed chronic strains of his neck, low back, right shoulder, and right knee. He made use of his military benefits to get some counseling though a local V.A. clinic. He presented himself as irritable, dejected, and intermittently tearful in our meeting.

Mike's story is one of an employee who incurred real injury as a result of an unsafe worksite. While there is an expectation that employers minimize hazards for their employees, this worker's injuries were largely the result of inattention to or neglect of basic safety measures. Mike's troubled marriage got worse with his injuries and loss of employment. The below-the-ground experience resulted in persistent fears, depression, and traumatic dreams. He ended up on an antidepressant for the first time in his life. He expected to settle his industrial injury claims and get by on Social Security Disability benefits. The only thing that gave Mike pleasure was going fishing at a nearby lake. Not a happy ending.

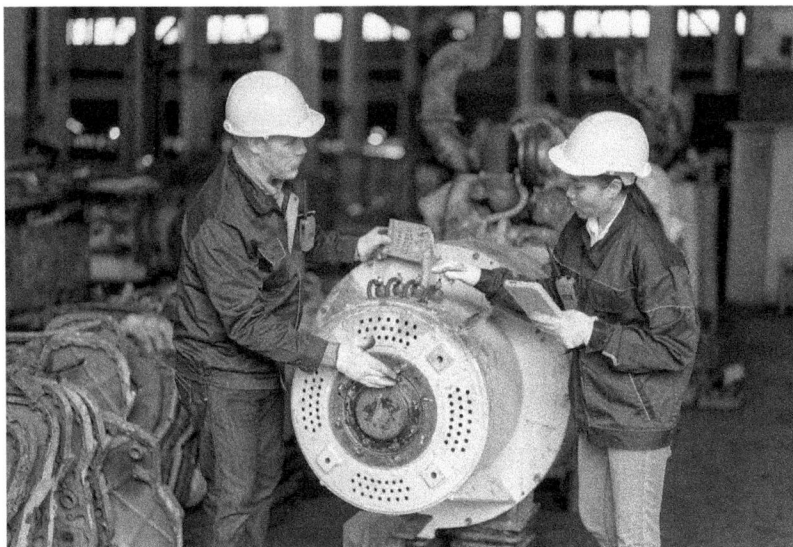

# 3  Maintenance Workers: Hurt by Equipment

## Maintenance Work Is Dangerous

The key to operating a safe worksite for maintenance workers is prevention. These workers are at risk from equipment, heights, electrical hazards, and the improper use of tools. Injury rates increase when safety procedures are ignored, hazards are not foreseen, machinery lockouts aren't used, improper use of ladders and scaffolding occur, and when electrical work is assumed by the untrained.[1]

## The Case of Sam Baron: Left with Limits

He was good with his hands and was talented when it came to troubleshooting. So, for ten years Sam Baron was the maintenance worker for an 80-unit apartment complex in a suburban community north of San Francisco. He did interior and exterior painting, appliance installation and repairs, patching of the complex's tar roofing, minor concrete fixes, and a variety of other tasks to keep up the structure of buildings beset by long-term wear and tear. Before coming to work at Shady Acres, Sam had spent six years providing maintenance services for another group of apartments in a neighboring community. He always thought he was appreciated by the owner for his common-sense approach to the needs of the residential tenants who were his responsibility.

Sam was using a dolly to move a replacement water heater up a ramp on the day he was hurt. He was working alone at the time. He could have used some assistance, but the tenants understandably wanted some hot water. He pushed and pulled on the dolly to get the large appliance into place. He was a bit tired when he gave one last tug to move the heater to the desired location. The acute low back and right leg pain was too intense for Sam to complete the task. He decided to rest before finishing the job that required repositioning the appliance to an upright position.

Sam and his wife lived on-site. He went to his apartment to take a break. His wife brought him an iced tea while he sat in a recliner. After half an hour, his pain was no better, and he couldn't get himself out of the chair without his wife's help. "Forget the water heater, Sam. I'm taking you to the E.R.," she told him. It was there he learned that he had herniated a disc in his lumbar spine while tearing the anterior cruciate ligament (ACL) in his right knee. The doctor on duty made it clear that Sam needed to be fixed. "I'm referring you to an orthopedist, giving you some meds for the pain, and taking you off work for the next few weeks." Those few weeks became months during which Sam received conflicting opinions about recommended treatment.

Sam came to regret his decision to install the appliance without assistance. That was how he rolled. He got things done. However, this time he faced serious consequences. Despite hoping that time would bring relief, that did not happen. He trusted the advice to have an arthroscopic procedure for the ACL tear that would remove the damaged tissue yet not reconstruct the ligament. He would get by with physical therapy to strengthen the muscles around that joint. The herniated disc wasn't going away, and a fusion procedure recommended by a neurosurgeon offered relief from the pain that radiated down his leg.

Sam was off work for more than eight months while he underwent the planned surgeries. He resumed his duties at the apartment complex with the permanent restriction of "no heavy lifting." He found himself welcomed back by tenants and management. His fears of being let go by his long-term employer dissipated, as did much of his emotional distress and disturbed sleep. "I guess my hard work made me valuable after all," he noted.

## The Case of Louie Van Ho: Unwelcome Changes

He was good at troubleshooting machinery. That's why Mr. Van Ho was recruited to take on the duties of a lead worker for Fix-It-Experts. Louie had been working for a competitor who didn't appreciate his skill set. Fix-It Experts wanted Louie's expertise. The work involved repairing mechanical systems for commercial office buildings and large residential housing complexes in Northern California.

Louie was thrilled by the offer he accepted, which included a decent salary increase, incentive pay, and the prospect to move into a supervisory role over time. Things went well for the first year with his new employer. He saw himself as proving he was up to the task while he became assured that he had made a good career move to join a team that was established and growing its client list.

While supervising the installation of a new HVAC system for an existing apartment building, Louie opted to join his company's work crew putting the replacement unit into its designated site. He was proving himself by not paying for an additional helper and getting the system functional in the time frame agreed upon, which avoided any late fees.

The low back pain started the evening Louie helped the crew muscle a new furnace into its planned site. What started out as a bad muscle strain turned out to be a lumbar disc herniation that resulted in a disc removal and insertion of an artificial disc. The pain didn't go away as expected. As his time off work became prolonged, Louie became dejected and worried. His fears were rooted in reality as he got notice of job termination when he was not found by his treating surgeon to be capable of the lifting requirements of his position.

At the age of thirty-one, Louie's life was dramatically altered by an injury that led to surgery, work restrictions, job loss, and the expectations that he would have to reinvent himself to become a knowledgeable worker who could not take on strenuous activities. His disability claim was resolved with a provision that he receive job retraining benefits. Like this man, how many of us are vulnerable to an unforeseen accident that requires us to adapt to survive?

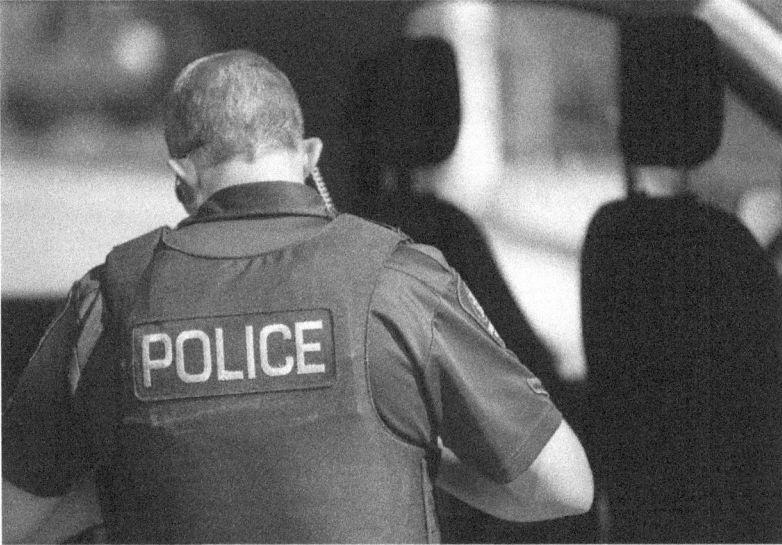

# 4   Police Officers: To Serve and Protect

## Officer Safety

An obvious form of physical violence for members of law enforcement in the U.S. is gun violence. Other physical risks include fights with offenders, vehicular pursuits, as well as equipment failure and fatigue.[1] Cops are also at risk for developing PTSD, depression, stress-related medical problems such as peptic ulcer disease and hypertension, and burnout (See discussion in Chapter 17).

## The Case of Detective Frank Robbins:
## A Career Confronting Violence

Frank Robbins came into my office and said, "I didn't grow up wanting to be a police officer." He was 52 years old, having joined the San Francisco Police Department in 1995. He worked as a plumber through college. Having grown up in the Bay area, he followed local teams and thought he might find a way to become a sportscaster. His bachelor's degree in communications from a private university did not open doors, as hoped for, in broadcasting. A co-worker at the plumbing company that employed them suggested applying to the police department in San Francisco. Two of his older brothers were cops. So, Frank became a cop.

By the time we met, Officer Robbins had walked the walk. He'd been on the front line. He'd seen his fair share of death. Years as a patrol officer led to his promotion to the rank of sergeant assigned to the Special Victims Unit dealing with domestic violence, financial crimes, elder abuse, and sexual assault. Frank was pretty sure he'd seen it all. His last assignment was as a homicide detective, which lasted almost a decade. He helped to catch some really bad guys. They included repeat offenders and gang-related murderers. He investigated a serial killer who was his victims' landlord. The few cases that could be proven had involved death by strangulation or poisoning. At the point that one perpetrator was convicted, he was believed to have been responsible for at least seven murders.

I met Sergeant Robbins through the Alternative Dispute Resolution program agreed to by management and the Police Officers' Union. For some time, he made use of alcohol to deal with the stress of investigating horrific crimes. He thought he could get through a few more years and then retire. Once he retired and no longer was exposed to more disturbing crime scenes, Frank figured he'd be better able to manage his drinking. It was his wife who made it clear that things had to change. The officer listened to her ultimatum of a marital separation if he didn't get help, so he entered a chemical dependency program with a good reputation. He became clean and sober while continuing to attend 12-step meetings.

Back at work, the officer remained a homicide detective. In fact, it turned out that he was an investigator of the mass shooting where I had evaluated thirteen victims. (See Chapter 19.) The shooter in that case was a driver with no prior history of significant violence or treatment for mental illness. He was an angry man who brought two handguns to work with the intention of shooting fellow employees. He killed three others before he killed himself. At least one co-worker was shot and survived. Many employees ended up needing time away from work. Several made use of mental health treatment to deal with intrusive recollections, traumatic dreams, and disturbed sleep that came forth as the result of that critical incident.

The workplace would never be the same for those who lived through it. The loss of life, the death claims brought by the families of the dead, and the workers' compensation claims for employees who survived had tainted the shipping hub. There was also a class action lawsuit brought against the security company that had allowed the shooter to sneak two weapons into what was expected to be a secure workplace. It was a notable event for Frank as well.

The officer began experiencing episodes of chest pain attributed to job stress. An initial cardiac workup found nothing worrisome. He remained abstinent from alcohol while continuing to investigate deaths attributable to murders. An episode of chest pain was so intense that he was taken to a local hospital where he underwent emergency stent placement to two coronary arteries. Apparently, there was a cardiovascular problem after all, which resulted in a myocardial infarction or heart attack.

That hospitalization led to a cumulative stress/trauma claim that culminated in Officer Robbins being evaluated by a cardiologist and Dr. Bob. His claims were accepted by his employer. The officer retired earlier than he expected. He stayed actively involved in his marriage and avocational interests such as golf. While remaining clean and sober, he preferred not to pursue counseling for the lingering anxiety related to far too many scenes of violence and death. His tale is just one example of the toll law enforcement can take upon those who pursue that line of work. Let us all be grateful there are cops and deputy sheriffs who serve and protect the rest of us.

## The Case of Officer John Dunst: Undercover Is Uncomfortable

Only in his 40s, he'd walked the walk, not just talked the talk. John Dunst became an officer in the California Highway Patrol after completing the CHP Academy at age twenty. He had shown his interest in law enforcement since he had gone on ride-alongs with cops as a teenager raised in a northern community of the San Francisco Bay. Prior to attending the academy, John had taken courses in criminal justice at the local community college. His initial assignment as a rookie cop was out of a South Bay office. He then transferred to a location closer to his residence in the North Bay. Unlike many of his peers, John was not particularly fond of traffic stops and other patrol duties. He made it clear he wanted to be impacting real crime.

John's interests were not lost on his commanding officer who recommended that a place be found for Officer Dunst with the California Department of Justice as a special agent. He worked out of a Central Valley office enforcing narcotics violations until he resigned from his job to stay home and care for his wife who was quite ill. After she had recuperated, John was reinstated by the CHP as a patrol officer for another year. He then became a detective on high-visibility cases dealing with sexual assaults, domestic violence, threats of public officials, and criminal conspiracy. By the mid-1990s, the CHP was being tasked with more law enforcement outside of the state's highways. Officer Dunst was assigned to a special investigative unit where he dealt with computer crimes, vehicular theft, cargo losses, and officer-involved shootings.

For five years, Officer Dunst worked undercover assignments where the officer's identity was unknown to most other police, sheriff's deputies, district attorneys, and judges in the region of California where he investigated organizations involved in "domestic terrorism." He infiltrated the Hell's Angels, the American Nazi Party, liberation parties for animal rights and the earth, communist party organizers, and other fringe groups with political agendas. His duties required him to have multiple identities at a given time. He participated in protests, demonstrations, and takeovers of corporate and government buildings. He was in deep.

Officer Dunst's home life suffered. His wife was put off by his attire, his body piercings, and his gruff demeanor. He distanced himself from colleagues, friends, neighbors, and family. Many who knew John could not easily relate to his undercover persona. His marriage didn't survive.

Work had taken this man to encampments of the Aryan Brotherhood, though he was raised in the Jewish faith. John was reassigned to an anti-terrorist unit at the Golden Gate Bridge. It was there he assisted in the recovery of the bodies of suicide victims. He also found himself identifying with animal rights protesters. His world made no sense, so he sought out help.

The good news is that John has retired, and he has the potential for a future. His case reminded me of Frank Serpico with the New York Police Department. Officer Serpico was a New

York cop, portrayed by Al Pacino in the 1973 film *Serpico*, who took enormous risks as an undercover officer. Sometimes, serious work has grave consequences. John Dunst survived his missions, but at what cost? If soldiers are recognized as having endured psychological scars from combat, should not our modern-day warriors on the home front be acknowledged for their sacrifice as well?

## The Case of Nancy Reeves: A Dramatic End to a Decade of Trauma

When Nancy Reeves came to work as a member of the Oakland Police Department, she was already serving as a reserve officer in the U.S. Army. She was the older of two daughters born to an African American couple who had been U.S. Marines. Nancy's parents' military service resulted in her family living in locations in the Midwest, Hawaii, and California during her childhood and adolescence. As a teenager it was apparent that Nancy was interested in other young women.

After receiving a bachelor's degree in business administration, Nancy went to work for a brokerage firm in the San Francisco Bay Area. She found the work unfulfilling, so she attended Officer Candidate School and joined the Army Reserves. Her next career move was to leave the field of business and complete the police academy for the City of Oakland. That led to assignments with Field Training Officers.

Officer Reeves proved to be a "hard charger" in her first two years assigned to patrol duties. Her police duties were at times interrupted by military service. She returned to a patrol assignment with the OPD with a promotion to sergeant. When she was asked to meet with me for a psychiatric evaluation, she was handling office duties as a captain in the Army Reserves. While submitting her application for a work-related disability retirement from law enforcement, she also expected to shortly complete her military obligation.

This officer's personnel file was teaming with notable events. Her patrol duties resulted in physical confrontations, shootings, car chases, and death scenes. She volunteered as a Black female officer for undercover assignments that proved to be demanding and stressful. She had witnessed victims of abdominal stab wounds, gunshot wounds to the chest, head injuries with visible brain matter, fatal hemorrhaging, and other adverse outcomes from acts of violence. She suffered through numerous critical incidents. This included shooting an armed suspect in the chest. He was treated and went to jail. She got some counseling.

It was a motor vehicle accident, while on duty, that could have taken Officer Reeves' life. While responding to a call, her police car was struck by a speeding drunk driver's vehicle. The police car was hit on the driver's side and careened across three lanes of traffic before it hit a tree. Officer Reeves was trapped with injuries to her left shoulder and knee. To her horror, a passerby leaned into the damaged car and fired a shot followed by two misfires. The officer could not access her weapon or a functioning radio. Physically hurt and terrified, it took several minutes, which felt like hours, before she was rescued by fellow officers who arrested the DUI suspect. Whoever fired the shot was long gone.

Why was the officer done with her police career? She had ongoing complaints related to injuries to the shoulder and knee that required surgery. The crash also resulted in chronic back pain. Intertwined with symptoms of depression and PTSD was a mild traumatic brain injury caused by the crash. I concurred with other doctors who advised against the sergeant returning to police duties. She was in physical pain, using various prescription drugs, had real musculoskeletal problems, and had lost her confidence to make command decisions. Once a hard charger, she was now a doubtful, slow ambler.

## The Case of Hans Schmidt: Haunted by Shootings

Officer Schmidt was the first member of his family to become a cop. He got involved in a youth program sponsored by a police department in Southern California. In his early twenties, he joined the Santa Barbara Police Department where he worked in patrol, vice, and gang unit assignments. He met and married a fellow officer. The couple decided to relocate after a female officer they knew was shot and killed. The officers ended up in a small town outside of Fresno. Hans later became a member of the Fresno Police Department.

Officer Schmidt was assigned duties as a field training officer, as a member of a tactical unit, and as a plainclothes officer investigating homicides and armed robberies. While he had never shot a suspect in Santa Barbara, the officer ended up in several officer-involved shootings in Fresno. His first involved a pizza parlor where the robber was shot and killed. Some months later, he shot a 19-year-old robbery suspect who survived. In a SWAT assignment, Hans shot and killed a perpetrator who had taken the life of a fellow officer. When assigned to a tactical unit, he shot and killed an armed suspect. On another occasion, he fatally shot a homicide suspect. His last shooting was of a single round that struck two thieves engaged in a vehicular theft. They survived.

Officer Schmidt was found to have acted properly in all these incidents. He was reluctant to discuss those events with his family. While treated for shingles, he learned there was a local psychologist who routinely counseled police experiencing PTSD following a critical incident. Officer Schmidt had participated in a number of those events. He also was told that his viral illness may have been triggered by stress. By the time he was seen through our offices, Hans was a man in his fifties and was struggling with neurologic and dermatologic symptoms related to a post-viral condition and from memories of trauma scenes.

My report recommended a small number of sessions to finish up with his psychologist and that this career officer receive a departmental commendation for his years of service. Many officers retire without shooting someone. Some officers are found to use lethal force unnecessarily. This officer made use of lethal force when necessary. He deserved some recognition for serving and protecting residents of a Central Valley city. Hans and his wife, who was retiring from her duties as an inspector, had plans to move to a more rural community known for its tranquility.

## The Case of Anna Stein: A Career Ended by Others

Anna Stein was accused of misconduct by two officers in her department's K-9 unit while on a trip to acquire new dogs for that specialized team. She had been recruited by a senior officer who knew her through her prior employment as an EMT in that Central Valley city's fire department. After completing six months of education in a police academy, she was given a patrol assignment. She was a patrol officer for two years before she became a member of a gang intervention unit. As she gained respect within the department, Officer Stein had a position created for her as a detective offering gang members "an alternative."

Anna had success in helping some members of a Latino gang give up their evil ways, so to speak. She made it apparent that they would be hounded if they continued their involvement in that multigenerational crime organization. After passing the sergeant's test, she was promoted and reassigned to patrol duties. Time seemed to fly by for Officer Stein, who had been with the department for ten years when she became a supervisor in the Mounted K-9 Unit. That required her to receive additional training in working with both police dogs and horses. The officer had no children of her own, so she came to view those animals as "my kids."

Sergeant Stein was not aware that there were members of her unit who resented her authority over them. She had not been a K-9 officer for that long when she was put in charge of the day shift. She also was considered bossy by her younger co-workers. It was because of the assignment to pick up a team of dogs that the sergeant learned there were allegations about her conduct during that week-long trip. Three officers claimed she had been drinking after the workday ended. Those co-workers each went to their captain upon returning from the business trip with an account of Officer Stein dancing around their bunkhouse in a provocative manner. They stuck to their stories that she had to be asked to go to her quarters.

An Internal Affairs investigation concluded that Officer Stein must have done what was alleged as those who complained consistently swore that she acted improperly. This led to disciplinary action that resulted in termination of her employment. She had been an officer heretofore with no blemishes on her record. After her dismissal, Anna hired an attorney. She had already been through a Skelly hearing where she pleaded her case to departmental administration. She filed a claim for psychiatric injury, better known as a stress claim. That's how we met.

My office issued a report that called into question the allegations of an officer in good standing. Apart from the personnel actions, Anna had a valid claim for symptoms of PTSD related to numerous critical incidents over the course of her career. It was left up to the trier of fact of the legal proceedings to determine whether the job termination was carried out in good faith though I suggested a more thorough investigation might have involved polygraphs, lie detector assessments, of her accusers. This case contrasts with the other tales in this chapter that chronicle the trauma that members of law enforcement routinely experience. Perhaps things have not changed so much in some situations for "the boys in blue." Would a male officer have lost his career for a single instance of foolish off-duty behavior?

*You may notice that this chapter has more cases than others in this collection of work-related tragedies and responses. Cops, sheriff's deputies, and other members of law enforcement have a special place among workers for me. I was a contract physician at Highland General Hospital for five years. Highland is the county hospital for Alameda County, east of San Francisco. All manner of mayhem comes to Highland. During my tenure in the early- to mid-1980s, that hospital had a busy medical E.R., a jail unit, and Psych Emergency Services, along with outpatient and inpatient services typical of an urban county hospital. There's not much opportunity for rest as a doctor on duty.*

*There were many occasions that an agitated patient or a troubled family member threatened me or others in my clinical team. I came to appreciate cops and deputy sheriffs who would intervene. They'd jump into harm's way. I owe these first responders some recognition and gratitude. These folks don't get paid enough to, literally, take the hits intended for others.*

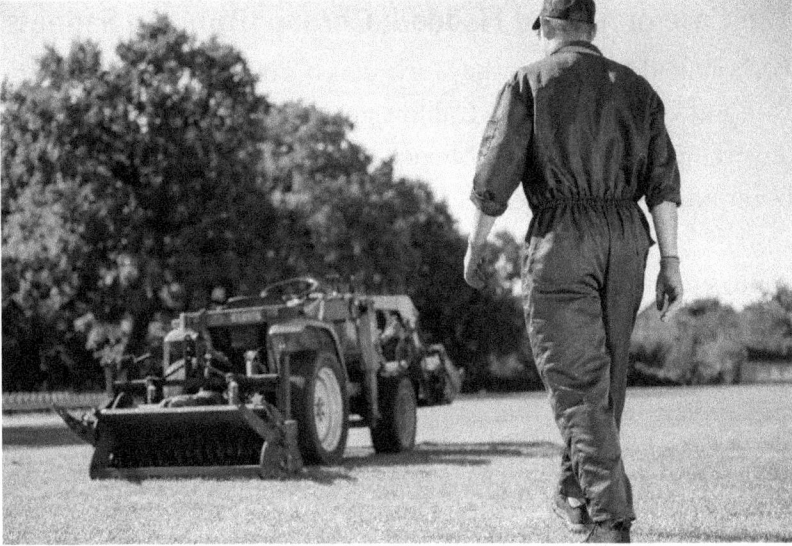

# 5    Grounds Maintenance Workers: Keeping Up the Outdoors

## The Hazards Associated with Work as a Groundskeeper

Groundskeepers risk a variety of physical injuries resulting from transportation incidents, contact with objects and equipment, falls, chemical exposure, electrocution, and weather conditions. More specifically, this includes tractor rollovers, motor vehicle accidents, being struck by tree limbs, being injured by power tools, herbicide poisoning, and prolonged high and low temperature exposure.[1]

## The Case of Ahmed Haddad: Chronic Pain and Sadness

For a half dozen years, he worked as a groundskeeper at a private golf club in Carmel, California. Ahmed Haddad grew up in a working-class family in Mexico where he worked as a farm laborer after finishing school. After coming to California, Ahmed worked in a packing shed, until being hired by a company that contracted to maintain the grounds at the golf course where he eventually was injured.

Ahmed's duties at Big Sur Links included mowing the lawns and greens, raking the sand traps, removing debris, and performing minor repairs and upkeep of the outdoor fixtures on the golf course. On the day he got hurt, he was using a faulty greens mower. It was a self-propelled mower that he guided from behind. When the mower suddenly lurched forward, he attempted to control the machine by pulling on it, but he lost his balance and fell backwards with his landing awkwardly on his buttocks. He recalls experiencing a "cracking" sensation in his low back. After a brief break, Ahmed worked for a few more hours before his acute pain led him to report the injury.

Ahmed was referred by his employer to a local urgent care clinic. The initial consultation included a brief physical examination and X-rays. He was in turn referred to an orthopedist who prescribed physical therapy, medication for pain and muscle spasms, and an MRI scan. That scan demonstrated a bulging disc at L4/5. After several months of treatment that included a series of epidural injections while away from his job duties, Ahmed agreed to undergo a discectomy. The surgery helped to the extent that he experienced less pain when walking. After obtaining legal representation, Ahmed came under the care of a physical medicine expert.

I evaluated Ahmed two years after his injury. He had recently returned to work at the golf club, where he was assigned work using a riding lawnmower. He was still treated with a mild

36

narcotic, an anti-inflammatory drug, and an antidepressant. He complained of constant low-back pain made worse by prolonged standing and cold weather. Conversely, the application of heat to his low back reduced muscle spasms and pain. He avoided heavy lifting.

The treatment records I reviewed described Ahmed as sad, frustrated, and tearful. Psychological test results were consistent with an individual who was depressed, anxious, and preoccupied with his physical health. A degree of symptom exaggeration of the test data was interpreted as a cry for help from a man who was struggling with feelings of hopelessness.

This worker's personal history included his being raised in rural Mexico where he attended public schools until he was fifteen. He then went to work as a farm worker while continuing to live in the family home. Ahmed was in his early twenties when he immigrated to the U.S. He and his female partner met while working on a farm near Salinas, California. The couple had been together for a dozen years and had two school-aged children. Aside from his work-related injury, Ahmed's medical history was unimpressive other than his having become abstinent from the use of alcohol following a DUI charge several years earlier. While he attended A.A. meetings in the past, he had never made use of counseling.

Ahmed was diagnosed as having a mood disorder or clinical depression associated with a chronic pain syndrome. His psychiatric symptoms of sadness, anxiety, frustration, and reduced hopefulness were the result of a compensable consequence psychiatric injury that was secondary to his admitted orthopedic injury. His relationship with his life partner was being challenged. The couple could benefit from professional help with how Ahmed's limitations were also affecting their life together. Along with a recommendation for treatment with another antidepressant that had greater efficacy for addressing pain and sleep issues, a short course of couple's therapy was in order.

Ahmed was going to lead his life differently due to the physical and mental impairment that would persist. I remember my mom saying, "We don't appreciate our health until we don't have it anymore."

## The Case of Hector Ruiz: A Shocking Experience

Hector Ruiz came to California from his homeland of Mexico as an adult and had a work history that involved jobs as a field worker, a gardener, and a handyman. When he immigrated to the Bay area from the coastal community of Zihuantanejo, Hector was guaranteed a job by his cousin who was a supervisor of a landscaping crew at a private Catholic college that was known, in part, for its Spanish-style architecture and pristine grounds.

After two years working at the college, Hector had proven himself as a dependable crew member who was good at troubleshooting irrigation systems, outdoor lighting, and pests and diseases affecting trees and shrubs. With the opening of a new library building on the school's campus, an accompanying landscaping plan that had a complex lighting component was conceived. In preparing for the new hardscaping, Hector was assigned the task of cutting through existing power lines that had been deactivated. He was told an electrician had tested the lines and had established that they could be removed. Using a power saw, Hector was cutting into the first of the lines when he was thrown back by the electrical charge of a circuit that was still hot.

Things had not added up in the medical work-up. Hector insisted the line that had shocked him carried 12,000 volts of electricity. There was no verification that was the case. His initial complaints included back pain, generalized weakness, and numbness in his left arm. A treating neurologist instituted treatment with antidepressant and antipsychotic drugs after describing exaggerated behavior on the part of his patient. An evaluating neurosurgeon documented unexplainable right-sided numbness and contrasting left-sided sensitivity to touch. Consideration was given to malingering or hysteria on Hector's part.

High-voltage electrical injuries are characterized by entry and exit wounds, cataract formation, and muscle damage affecting the heart. Instead, Hector complained of muscle pain and weakness that resulted in his using a cane to move about. Of some importance to his dramatic presentation was his background that involved minimal contact with the healthcare system, predating his work-related incident. He insisted that a doctor at a county clinic had told him he would never recover from the shock that could have killed him. Psychological testing conducted through our office was consistent with a person who was preoccupied with his physical health while reporting symptoms of anxiety, depression, and auditory hallucinations.

Referrals for pain management services and psychotherapy had been ineffective in reducing Hector's physical complaints or his emotional distress. He insisted the "black spots" he now saw had never been there in the past. No reassurance from an ophthalmologist that the spots were benign vitreous floaters that are commonly experienced and have no relationship to the electrical shock assuaged Hector's fears that he had been severely damaged.

I recommended an alternative position for Hector at the college that had nothing to do with electrical wiring. No further medication trials nor counseling sessions were likely to change his psychosomatic array of dysfunction. Chronic sprains had morphed into a life-altering set of self-imposed restrictions for this unsophisticated, vulnerable employee. For Hector to continue with landscaping work, his fears would have to be accommodated such that he could be assured that co-workers would handle any electrical tasks in the future. This tale is an example of how a life event can precipitate a specific phobia, i.e. electrophobia, or the irrational fear of electricity and electrical devices. More common specific phobias include fear of spiders, snakes, heights, dogs, and agoraphobia or the fear of open spaces and crowded situations.

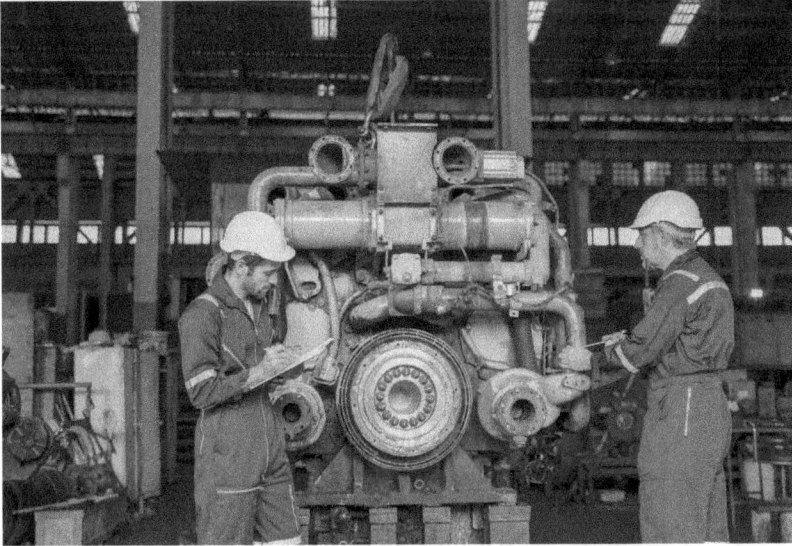

# 6 Heavy Equipment Mechanics: Working on Big Stuff

## Fixing Big Stuff Is Risky

One need not have much imagination to understand the risks associated with servicing and repairing big machinery. It's easy to get hurt. According to the online publication *Occupational Safety & Health,* the main risks in working with heavy equipment are operating machinery without proper guards, risky behavior resulting in crushes and run-overs, accidents while transporting equipment, inadequate communications regarding hazards, and inadequate safety training.[1]

## The Case of Ricky Gomez: Living with Localized Pain

Ricky Gomez was used to working on a ranch because he grew up on one outside of Mexicali, Mexico. He was one of twelve children. His dad was a farmer and rancher who grew crops such as cotton, wheat, and barley, in addition to raising livestock for the family's consumption. Ricky was expected to do chores from an early age. He attended a local school through the seventh grade, at which point he worked as a ranch hand in the family business. At eighteen, Ricky came to Los Angeles with his girlfriend. They both worked picking strawberries. The big city was not to Ricky's liking, so the couple moved to a small town outside of Fresno.

The couple married while Ricky stayed employed as a farm worker until he was hired as an equipment mechanic by Hanley Equipment Services. He learned to work on tractors, trucks, and harvesters from his father. The company owner, Art Hanley, observed Ricky troubleshooting some farming equipment and hired him on the spot. For the next fifteen years, Ricky was a mechanic who performed maintenance and repairs on all manner of machinery and heavy equipment used on a 40,000-acre ranch, in part operated by Hanley Equipment. Ricky enjoyed the work and felt respected by the owner and co-workers. After his marriage ended, he shared custody of his three kids with his ex-wife. Sometime later, he divorced his second wife, though there were no children involved. He stayed living in the same home and decided to remain single.

While disconnecting a trailer from the hitch of a company pickup truck, Ricky's left, dominant hand was crushed. He was rushed to an E.R., where a determination was made that a hand surgeon was needed. Surgery was performed at a university medical center for a fractured metacarpal requiring hardware to stabilize a broken bone in his hand. The surgeon also addressed soft tissue damage during that procedure. Even with the passage of time and a course of physical therapy, Ricky complained of unrelenting pain and reduced grip strength in the affected hand. The treating surgeon documented the presence of contractures and scarring that complicated the healing process. A consulting neurologist diagnosed reflex sympathetic dystrophy, also known as a complex regional pain syndrome. The neurologist made changes to Ricky's medication to address his pain.

I met with Ricky fifteen months after the crush injury occurred. He complained of hand pain made worse by activity. His pain would wake him while he slept fitfully. Apart from his physical symptoms, Ricky was sad, worried, and frustrated. He needed his hand fixed to return to work and have some semblance of a normal life. His psychological test results were consistent with a man struggling with depression, anxious worry, and diminished hopefulness about his future. My assessment was that Ricky was experiencing an expected adjustment disorder to a bona fide stressor. I recommended a particular antidepressant that could address pain and disturbed sleep, along with his emotional distress.

More importantly, I concurred with a consulting orthopedist who recommended treatment with anti-inflammatory medication and cortisone injections. A crush injury can result in physical disability and a prolonged clinical depression. In Ricky's case the input of various clinicians allowed for sufficient improvement that he regained enough of his pre-injury capacity to perform his mechanic's duties, albeit with some struggle on his part.

## The Case of Henry Fairbanks:
## The Power of Heavy Equipment

Henry Fairbanks came to the job as an experienced mechanic. He enjoyed his time with Bay Piping, working out of a location on the Sacramento River, southwest of the city of Sacramento and northeast of San Francisco.

Henry was a whiz with diesel engines. He could also service and repair brake systems, transmissions, suspensions, as well as tires and wheels. H.F., as he was known to the team at Bay Piping, fixed trucks, trailers, drilling rigs, and all the heavy equipment needed by a company known for drilling wells, operating oil derricks, and laying pipe to move all types of liquid matter. He earned his pay and bonuses.

What brought Henry to meet with me was an accident, an unusual occurrence, a blow-up. Literally, a blow-up.

Henry was filling a tire on one of the company's forklifts when the metal rim exploded. Henry placed a rag on the right side of his face while remaining conscious though dazed. He called out for help. His injuries were initially assessed at a local community hospital before he was transferred to a trauma center. After he was stabilized, Henry underwent right wrist surgery. He was left with permanent blindness in his right eye, post-traumatic headaches, and persistent pain throughout much of his right side due to sprains attributed to the exploding rim.

A mild post-traumatic brain injury had left this worker with cognitive deficits affecting his short-term memory. This was made worse by his becoming depressed for the first time in his life. To deal with the headaches and pain, he made use of anticonvulsant and antidepressant medication that left him drowsy. Henry became sensitive about his appearance as he was left with gruesome scars across his face. He had yet to meet with a plastic surgeon when I interviewed him via Zoom software during the COVID-19 pandemic. By then, he had become reclusive while recuperating at home.

My recommendations included having a primary treating physician take charge of Henry's care. He needed a consultation with a skilled cosmetic surgeon. He needed to be offered individual psychotherapy. He might also benefit from trials of other antidepressants for his persistent depression. These elements of treatment should already have been in place.

This was a serious set of injuries, yet no CalOSHA investigation had taken place. Henry had yet to be evaluated by a vocational counselor for potential retraining. He was being allowed to languish. The employer and its insurer were due penalties for maintaining an unsafe workplace. I was outraged that H.F. was not receiving coordinated medical treatment.

It is in cases such as that of Henry Fairbanks that we are reminded of how a single event can alter one's life. This man's worksite was not known for being unsafe. Even when proper measures are taken to prevent injuries, malfunctions can occur. Of course, that was little solace for a man who would be left with significant physical and psychological wounds. Some work has inherent dangers.

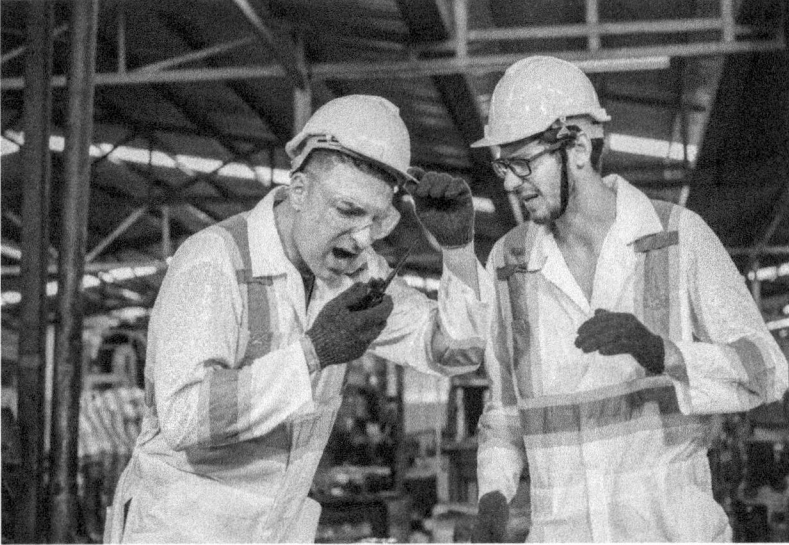

# 7   Supervisors Of Mechanics: Workplace Conflict

## Many Who Supervise Mechanics Regret It

**B**eing the supervisor or foreman of maintenance mechanics requires a variety of skills. Expertise begins with preventative maintenance. In a modern worksite, familiarity with computer systems to organize and manage work orders is necessary. Supervisors must ensure that equipment is maintained so that troubleshooting and operations function properly. These same supervisors will oversee plumbing and HVAC systems. Plant safety is a priority for these foremen. Improvement in procedures, operations planning, and plant maintenance become the responsibility of these supervisors. A program, including standards, for equipment such as ladders and cranes, is all part of these workers' duties.[1]

Supervisors who manage mechanics must be prepared for conflict, including disagreements over work processes, interpersonal tension, and differing opinions.[2] So, mechanics' supervisors are at risk for physical injury related to worksite hazards along with the potential for interpersonal conflict, including physical violence, when disagreements arise.

## The Case of Tony Genoa: Working for a Bad Boss

Tony Genoa was a skilled mechanic who learned the trade from his father while growing up in Colorado. After graduating from high school, Tony enlisted in the U.S. Marine Corps where his primary duties involved his servicing vehicles for a combat unit. After receiving an honorable discharge, the ex-Marine returned to Colorado with a wife and young child. He was kept busy as a truck mechanic though his marriage suffered. Some time went by before his wife opted for divorce. Tony remarried that year and moved with his new bride to California.

With his wealth of experience, Tony found a job as a mechanic at Napa Motor Sales. He quickly became the lead mechanic, and in his early thirties he oversaw a young crew. The company bought and sold used cars and trucks. Tony had responsibility for approving purchases of vehicles. He even took on sales work when needed. He reported directly to the owner.

For three years, Tony did as he was instructed by his boss. Yet he felt trapped by having purchased a pickup truck from the owner which was taking time to pay off. However, it was other aspects of the job that wore on Tony. He agreed to roll back the odometer on a luxury sedan with high mileage, only to learn that the company owner expected that type of fraud to be part of the job. Tony also resented the long work hours without receiving overtime pay.

Tony was directed to replace the engine on a vehicle without having the assistance of a helper or the proper equipment. Working alone, he lifted too much, which led to him being treated for an upper back and neck strain. While his musculoskeletal symptoms gradually improved, he reinjured himself when pulling on an overhead door at the shop. His treating physician placed restrictions on this worker's activities. The shop owner ignored those restrictions.

Later a suspicious fire at the worksite destroyed all the records in the business office. Tony became convinced the fire was not accidental. The business was closed and none of the workers got any severance pay. When filing for unemployment benefits, Tony learned that his boss was in arrears on payroll taxes. After turning back odometers, being needlessly injured, having his medical advice ignored, and the shop closing due to a suspicious fire, Tony's struggle to receive unemployment benefits was the last straw. He filed claims for physical and mental injury. He also cooperated with a criminal investigation of his employer's business practices.

Tony's orthopedic injuries improved with time and chiropractic treatment. He found a new job as the lead mechanic for a reputable shop and vowed to never again be coaxed into questionable or illegal practices. He considered his experience at the shuttered business to have been a painful learning lesson as it had financial and legal ramifications for Tony.

## The Case of Jose Aquino: Why Can't We Get Along?

Twenty years ago, Jose Aquino began working for MUNI, the transit system in San Francisco. He had immigrated from the Philippines where he had been a skilled mechanic. Jose had fam-

49

ily in the Bay area. In fact, he lived with some of his cousins. At the workplace, his knowledge about the mechanical systems of buses led to him being promoted to a lead position. That did not sit right with everyone. Five years into his employment, Jose directed another mechanic to check the brakes on a bus in the shop.

Jose's interactions with others were often perceived as odd. He was good with machines and less so in social situations. When directed to the task at hand, a worker he supervised took that action as punishment, especially after Jose made a joke with another employee. That action was perceived as having evil intent. The worker assaulted Jose with a screwdriver, causing abrasions and minor lacerations. At the county hospital, Jose received a few stitches; there was no need for surgery.

His assailant was terminated from employment, but Jose remained on a disability leave for two years following the workplace assault. He was treated by several physicians for musculoskeletal complaints with various medications, including opioid analgesics. Symptoms of anxiety, depression, and post-traumatic stress were emphasized by virtually all doctors who consulted on this worker's case. When his treating psychiatrist released Jose to return to his lower-level supervisory position, he took on those duties without difficulty.

Fifteen years after the assault, I was asked to evaluate Jose, as his claim for physical and mental injury had never been resolved. Doctors provided a confusing array of opinions. A police detective had concluded there was insufficient evidence to file charges of assault as Jose was described as having engaged in mutually combative behavior. His workers' comp claim was closed out with the stipulation that he have access to follow-up care with his former psychiatrist. Whatever took place at the worksite was colored by Jose's odd demeanor and mistrust of people in general. After years of clinical intervention for which there was little agreement among the doctors, more issues seemed unanswered than answered. There was no reason to believe further diagnostic testing or trials of drugs would bring clarity about what troubled this man. In some cases, victims of workplace trauma and violence may have contributed to the problematic interpersonal behavior. A doctor's ability to bring forth a pleasing resolution to those involved in the conflict is often quite limited.

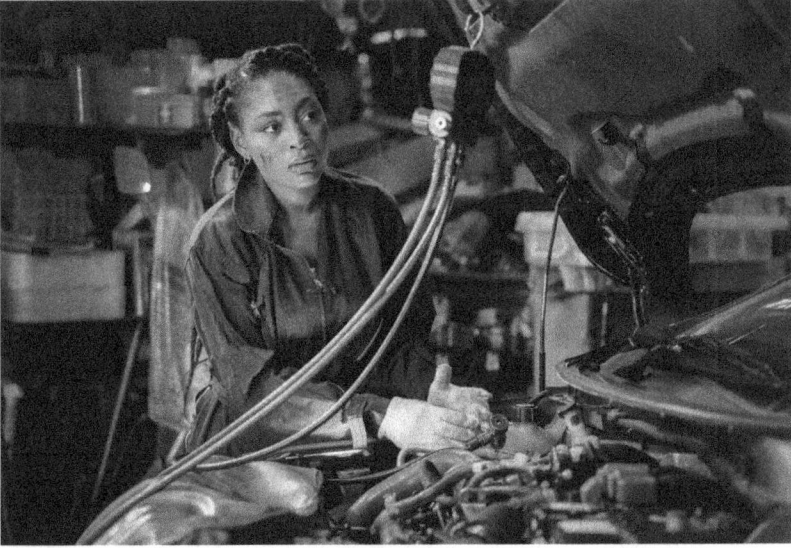

# 8    Small-Engine Mechanics: Accidents Happen

## What Hazards Are Common with Small Engines?

**Mechanics who work on small engines perform** maintenance, testing, and repairs of various forms of equipment that include motorcycles, motorboats, lawn mowers, and other equipment that use combustion engines.[1] Adequate ventilation is important when working on small gasoline engines. Workers can easily prevent carbon monoxide poisoning by working with engines operating in open spaces with adequate ventilation.[2] Because these workers address other mechanical features of equipment beyond engines, there are other physical injuries they may encounter.

## The Case of Darren Goodfellow: A Nice Ending for a Good Fellow

He'd worked on motorcycles, lawn mowers, and various 2-cycle engines over the previous decade. He got things done, until he couldn't. Darren Goodfellow was darn good at implementing common sense solutions to keep machinery functional. A buddy recruited this experienced mechanic to come to work for Hayward Harley-Davidson around the time there was a change in ownership. The business had a loyal customer base because of fair prices on sales of new and used bikes. The shop serviced and repaired all makes and models of Harleys dating back to one of the original V-twin engines reportedly manufactured in 1909.

Darren was thrilled to work in a quality shop. One year into his employment at Hayward H-D, he proclaimed to his wife, "Baby, I'm like a pig in shit." As the years went by, he stayed healthy until he felt a popping sensation when reaching overhead for a wrench that was laying on a high shelf. During a one-month medical leave recommended by his regular doctor, he took it easy. He returned to work and got by taking an occasional over-the-counter anti-inflammatory drug when he felt soreness in his low back.

A few years after his minor back injury, Darren experienced a new popping sensation when lifting and turning while holding a tire and rim assembly he was replacing. This time, he hurt his neck. His employer made an appointment at a local occupational medicine clinic that recommended radiologic studies, a trial of a muscle relaxant, and a pain management consultation. Epidural steroid injections worked for a time. Darren was also reassigned to counter duties where he wrote up repair orders for customers. Those light duties allowed for his pain to subside. Yet it was dealing with customers and the service manager that got to him.

Another year went by while Darren continued to work as a service advisor. He was provided with an ergonomic chair and workstation that seemed to help. He occasionally took a prescription narcotic when the neck pain was intense. It was due to a heated argument involving a new mechanic and a complaining customer that Darren began hyperventilating. He returned to the occupational medicine clinic where he was given anti-anxiety medication. After bringing the recent developments to the service manager's attention, he was told he needed to toughen up.

Darren felt trapped. He wasn't healthy enough to return to his mechanic's duties, and he knew he couldn't expect support from his manager. So, Darren contacted the insurance company representative assigned to his workers' comp claim. He was surprised to learn he had a right to vocational rehabilitation.

In his fifties, Darren began taking coursework in computer technology at a local community college where he was one of the oldest students. He did well academically in his first term. At that point, one of his instructors arranged a meeting with the dean of the college. That meeting led to a job offer for this injured mechanic to become the newest member of the faculty in the school's industrial arts program. Teaching the next generation of mechanics, avoiding strenuous activities, and being in a minimally stressful workplace did the trick. The faculty and students appreciated Darren. His chronic pain improved to the point he no longer made use of pain medication. His use of the anti-anxiety drug ended as well. This former mechanic eventually retired after ten years of teaching. At his retirement party, he was presented with a gold-plated wrench by a group of grateful students.

## The Case of Ronald James: A Series of Injuries

At the point Ronald James and I met, he was a man in his mid-fifties who had consulted with specialists in orthopedics, pain management, psychology, psychiatry, addiction medicine, and the list goes on. He had qualified for Social Security Disability benefits. A neurosurgeon had fused two vertebrae in his cervical spine, leaving him with stabilizing hardware in his neck. Scans of his lumbar spine demonstrated degenerative disc disease, bulging discs, and nerve impingement at multiple levels of his spine in his low back.

Ronald's saga with pain, numbness, disturbed sleep, irritability, and depression dated back more than ten years. After leaving the Army as a young adult, Ronald went to work at a motorcycle shop where he serviced transmissions, clutches, brakes, tires and wheels, shock absorbers, and engines. He had gained some experience as a mechanic during his time in the military. Ronald lived in several communities in the Midwest before he and his wife of several years relocated to northern California. He always found work at motorcycle dealerships and repair shops. With time, he became the old man who was relied upon by fellow mechanics.

In 1996, Ronald was working in a repair shop specializing in BMW motorcycles. He slipped on spilled oil while carrying a gas tank, landing on his back and striking his head the concrete floor of the repair shop. After months of treatment with medication, injections, and physical therapy, Ronald opted for surgery to address a disc herniation in his neck. A lengthy period of recovery followed.

Ronald was told it was safe to return to his mechanical work if he avoided heavy lifting. While his job experience was attractive to prospective employers, his lifting limits were not. A series of jobs followed, but either his employers didn't want to accommodate his limitations or he was too concerned that he would get hurt again.

While working for yet another motorcycle shop, Ronald lifted a heavy parts order and immediately knew he had made a mistake. This time it was an injury to his low back or lumbar spine that was the issue. Time away from heavy work activities seemed to help. Ronald received physical therapy and avoided an invasive procedure.

At a point where his pain was in control, Ronald took a job as a shop supervisor. Things went well enough that he was getting by with much less medication. That was until he drove to a convention with the owner of the shop where he worked. The journey was longer than expected, and Ronald needed help getting out of the passenger's seat of his boss' fancy pickup. After the convention, he rode home in that same vehicle. A consultation with his former surgeon produced new concern over a low back "that's a wreck."

Upon the advice of a former surgeon, Ronald sought treatment from a physician who specialized in managing chronic pain. By this point, he was receiving temporary disability benefits for a new work-related injury. When those benefits were exhausted, Ronald took a job as a security guard. Work as a mechanic, even on small engines, could result in the need for an invasive procedure to his low back.

Despite being proud of working for a living, after a few months providing security services, Ronald gave up and followed the advice he had been given to file for Social Security benefits. He qualified for such, but he still struggled financially to make ends meet. His wife was still employed at a preschool, and their daughter had work as a nanny. The attorney who had represented Ronald on the 1996 injury agreed to reopen his case with new injuries being the responsibility of subsequent employers.

When I met this now ex-mechanic, he came across as miserable. His clinical file included records and reports from dozens of doctors, four deposition transcripts of the injured worker related to multiple employers, and other administrative files related to claims with insurers and government agencies. Yuck! It was not difficult to feel empathy for Ronald's plight. He was leading a very restricted existence. Aside from over-the-counter medications, he was regularly making use of two narcotic analgesics, an anticonvulsant, two antidepressants, a mood stabilizer, a muscle relaxant, a drug to induce sleep, and a psychostimulant to counter the sedating effect of the other drugs.

My advice was to reduce the complexity of this man's drug regimen. Adding more drugs had increased the likelihood of drug interactions, side effects, and additive effects. Remember, do no harm. I also recommended that he discontinue meeting with a psychologist who was asking Ronald to go back through prior life traumas. He was given additional disability benefits as an acknowledgment of his depression and worry.

In the case of Ronald James, we see a worker with cumulative physical injuries that take a toll upon his well-being while having an adverse effect upon his psyche. Sometimes the damage done cannot be undone.

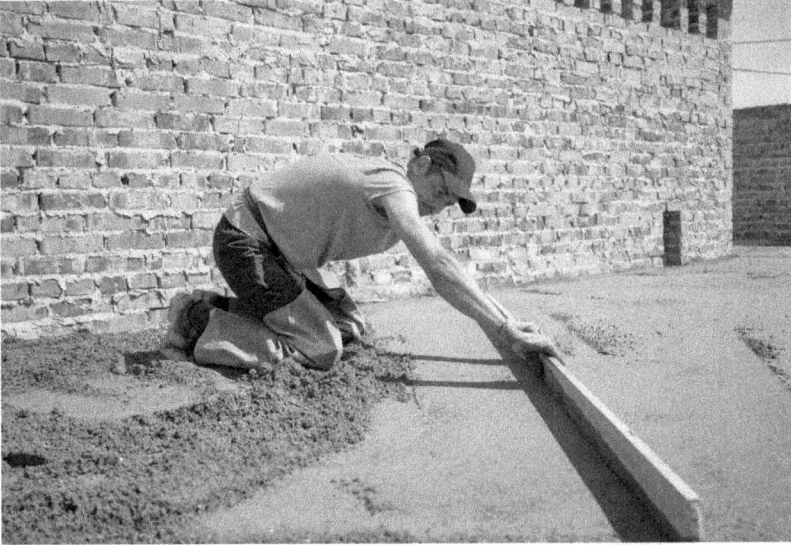

# 9 Cement Masons: Trips, Slips, and Falls

## What Dangers Befall Those Working with Concrete?

Masons use cement, bricks, cement blocks, and natural and manufactured stone to build structures. Masons make on average about $50,000 annually.[1] Common injuries result from heavy falling objects; trips, falls, and slips; electrical shocks; excavations or cave-ins; walls that give way or collapse; objects with sharp edges or protrusions; contact with high temperatures; and exposure to toxic substances.

## The Case of Jonny Rodriguez:
## Incidental Findings and Unfounded Complaints

Jonny Rodriguez had worked for the construction company for only a few months when he had to set aside his duties as a cement mason. Jonny was an experienced cement mason in his early fifties when he came to work for Jones Construction in 2012. Jonny operated his own small business as a self-employed cement contractor for years until a downturn in the economy caused him to shut things down. He then spent a couple of years as a hardware store employee. With the construction industry in California's Central Valley becoming vibrant once again, Jonny was glad to be back at the work he was good at performing.

Jones Construction worked on medium-size construction projects such as new schools and highways. On the date he was injured, Jonny was part of a crew working on an expansion of a Chevy dealership outside of Fresno. His job was, in part, to prepare the site for footings, which required him to set rebar in trenches with concrete. A pickup truck came through the site, and its driver was unaware that there were workers standing, sitting, or bending over in trenches while doing their jobs. Jonny was hit by the vehicle and briefly lost consciousness. Co-workers pulled him back to ground level with the pickup having gotten stuck in that trench.

Before he was taken to a local hospital by paramedics, the cement mason heard an EMT say, "Be careful with this guy, he could be paralyzed." At the hospital, Jonny started to regain sensation in his legs. He was told he had experienced a concussion and would need to give his body time to heal. We met one year later.

Jonny reported that while in the hospital he was told, "Your brain got rattled." That didn't sound too bad at the time. After several days as an inpatient, Jonny went home with outpatient care assigned to a physiatrist, or a physical medicine specialist. The "wounded" worker was hurting in his head, neck, and throughout his back. While away from this job, Jonny met with a physical therapist who was encouraging. Jonny took pills as needed for pain, muscle spasms, and insomnia. He had no union representation, but another Jones Construction employee made sure that a workers' comp claim was filed for Jonny. He was grateful to receive a check every two weeks when unable to return to work.

Something commonly happens when we undergo a thorough medical evaluation. Physicians can discover pathology unrelated to the injury. Doctors refer to these matters as "incidental findings." Incidental to whom? For Jonny to be told he had cardiovascular issues that were not due to his industrial injuries caused him worry. How could he pay for treatment of health problems that his company's insurer determined to be pre-existing?

When we met, Jonny was awaiting decisions about recommended medical care. A consulting orthopedist recommended arthroscopic surgeries for both shoulders. Jonny was willing to do whatever it took to get back to work. He was convinced that his cardiac problem was due to the stress of having been injured at work. He complained of unrelenting pain and neurologic symptoms such as intermittent muscle weakness that caused him to drop things or require that he rest on the floor. While it is possible for nerve damage, muscle spasms, and chronic sprains to result from the type of insult that Jonny had, extensive testing did not confirm there was an anatomical or physiologic basis for his wide-ranging symptoms and complaints.

Jonny's psychological test results were consistent with his having concerns about his health, complaining of profound depressive symptoms, and being exceedingly pessimistic about his future. Additional sources of information were requested to better establish how seriously injured Jonny was soon after the injury event. Facts make a difference. In my role as a consulting psychiatrist, I cautioned those involved in the care of this worker to avoid invasive procedures, the "off label" use of prescription drugs, and performing unnecessary testing. There are other explanations for cases of prolonged recovery and nonphysiologic symptoms other than the term "malingerer."

Other explanations for Jonny's clinical presentation included a psychosomatic condition, a somatoform disorder, and fibromyalgia. In an unsophisticated person prone toward developing unfounded symptoms and complaints, sometimes doing less is the prudent course to take. Even so, the overall prognosis in Jonny's case, given his industrial orthopedic problems, his nonindustrial cardiovascular issues, and tendency to develop psychosomatic complaints, made it unlikely that he could persist in assuming heavy labor activities for the long-term.

## The Case of Alberto Florio:
## Hard Hats Make a Difference

Alberto Florio came to live with his father in California from his homeland of El Salvador when he was sixteen. He was from a family of eight children raised in a ranch setting. He had little formal education. His father helped Alberto get a job with his employer, a landscaping company in a town outside of San Jose, California. After a couple of years work as a laborer, this young man was hired by a concrete contractor engaged in new residential construction projects. For the next few years, he learned how to build foundations, retaining walls, as well as walkways and driveways. He was a helper working with cement masons.

As a man in his early twenties, Alberto had been with Rock Hard Construction for only a few months when he was injured. The company had an expertise in reinforcing and replacing existing building foundations in locations in the southern end of the San Francisco Bay area. Alberto's job was to put into place

62

wooden forms for the pouring of concrete under existing homes. As he was quite slim, "the kid," as he was nicknamed by his crew, could move through crawl spaces with ease.

On the date of injury, Alberto was working under a home with about an 18-inch clearance between the ground and the first floor's substructure. Turning quickly in response to some instructions from the crew chief, this worker struck the right frontal side of his head against a metal pipe. He felt a bit dazed when he crawled out from beneath the house. He had not been wearing a hard hat. While taking a break and getting a drink of water, a right-sided headache became noticeable and increasingly intense. Given that Alberto could not stand up without swaying, his co-workers knew something was wrong. He was helped into the company pickup truck and taken to a nearby E.R.

It turned out that Alberto had an intracerebral hemorrhage or brain bleed. It was later determined, when he underwent emergency neurosurgery, that he had a pre-existing vascular malformation that had never been recognized. A large hematoma or blood clot was evacuated from an area of his frontal and temporal lobes of the brain. The patient was discharged after more than two weeks, only to be readmitted when persistent headaches, vertigo or a spinning sensation, and loss of his left field of vision required further investigation. Remnants of the vascular malformation were precisely removed during a craniotomy procedure performed by a highly skilled surgeon.

Not surprisingly, Alberto experienced sadness and worry while recuperating from treatment. The surgeries had prevented further damage, yet he was left with headaches, dizziness, limited vision, and problems with his balance. He was advised to forego his participation in recreational soccer. His medication regimen included an anti-inflammatory drug, an antihistamine for vertigo, and an antidepressant. His partial loss of vision could not be corrected. He was living with other family members while considering a return to El Salvador to help in a shop owned by his mother's family.

I recommended continued use of the antidepressant and some counseling while Alberto would be making decisions about his future. The hemorrhage had not occurred absent the blow to the head though Alberto may have been at risk for an unrelated problem had he not had the surgeries. The consulting physicians agreed that use of a protective hardhat would have prevented an injury that could have been catastrophic. A principle of occupational medicine and public safety involves the expectation that an employer will maintain reasonable safety measures to minimize accidents and injuries. This follows from the phrase attributed to Benjamin Franklin, "An ounce of prevention is worth a pound of cure." The pre-existing condition and the inattention on the employer's part to a basic safety measure complicated the issue of liability and ultimately delayed treatment in this worker's case.

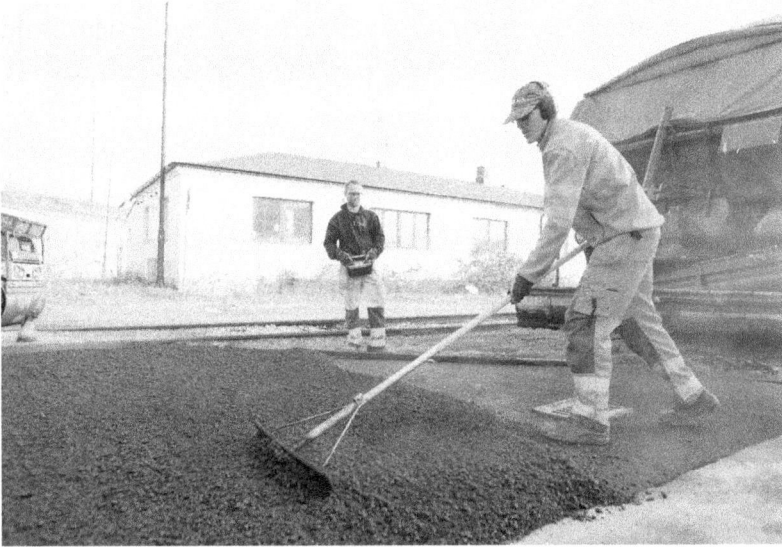

# 10 Highway Maintenance Workers: Lethal Hits

## Highway Maintenance Workers: Stay Vigilant

Weather, car crashes, and heavy traffic along roads, streets, and bridges wear out the pavement, the signage, and the supportive structures along a given roadway, so they will always need maintenance. Potholes need to filled. Lighting needs to be improved. Dead limbs need to be removed.

Highway work zones are hazardous because of vehicular movement through an area where maintenance and repairs are being made to a road surface and its adjoining structures, e.g., curbs, drainage, signage. Along with traffic passing through, there are often construction vehicles, heavy equipment, and power tools in use. Drivers must pay attention to signs, barrels, and lane changes. Fatal worker events are in large part the result of an individual being struck by a vehicle. According to the National Institutes of Occupational Safety and Health, for the timeframe of 2011–2018, the types of vehicles commonly causing worker deaths at these work zones were, in descending order, pickups and SUVs, automobiles, machinery, semi-trucks, and dump trucks.[1]

## The Near Fatal Crash of Tom Paris: Don't Drink and Drive

Tom Paris was in his late fifties when he and I met after he had been injured at work one too many times. Tom had been working in highway construction and maintenance throughout his adult life. He had been a valued employee of Sacramento Road Warriors for three decades. He thought he had seen it all. He had used asphalt to patch potholes. He had directed traffic as a flagman. There was a period of a few years when he operated a paving machine. He had incurred a work-related lifting injury, years earlier. His orthopedist agreed with his claim of cumulative trauma resulting in degenerative disc disease in his low back. Despite the sprains and strains that came and went, Tom didn't take much time away from work because he considered himself to be a "road warrior."

That all changed on a date four years earlier when Tom was operating the company street sweeper in preparation for his crew making some needed repairs to a stretch of a rural highway in the Sacramento River Delta. It was around 2 a.m. when "I knew I had been rear-ended." A powerful SUV slammed into the sweeper, which in turn left the highway before it came to rest against a large Oak tree. "I thought I was gonna burn to death,"

Tom reported. The other driver was a woman who had minor injuries to her face. She was arrested on the scene as it was determined she met the criteria for DUI violation with a Breathalyzer test of 0.20% blood alcohol content. She had been drinking with friends at a local bar for hours until closing time.

Meanwhile, it took two hours for a firefighting crew to extract Tom from the cab of the sweeper where he ended up crammed against the vehicle's steering wheel. That model was not equipped with an airbag. "The smell of diesel fuel scared the hell out of me. Thank God, one of the firefighters cut the electrical system," he said. Once extricated from the wrecked sweeper, the worker was taken to a local trauma center where his acute injuries were assessed.

Tom underwent multiple surgeries to repair an open fracture of his left tibia and a left knee with torn tendons and ligaments. A lengthy period of rehabilitation followed during which he had to learn to walk again. His twenty-eight years of employment with the company ended, and he became eligible to receive disability benefits.

Following the work-related accident, Tom lived with two adult sons who were employed and volunteered to help their father out while he recovered from his multiple injuries. Those sons were the product of his second marriage. He raised all four of the offspring after their mother essentially abandoned them. For his chronic pain, Tom was using fentanyl on a regular basis. He had never been treated for mental problems in the past, but he did see a psychologist while hospitalized for his left leg injuries and a mild concussion.

Tom wanted to close the chapter on this incident that had changed his life. His neuromusculoskeletal problems had stabilized. No further surgery was contemplated. I recommended he be referred to a pain management specialist with the intention of weaning him off narcotic medication while substituting alternatives that were not addictive. It was also recommended that the antidepressant duloxetine replace the psychotropic drug prescribed by his primary care physician following the accident. This was also a better choice for addressing pain and depression. The workers' compensation insurer paid the cost for support from a psychologist while Tom was transitioning to a new lifestyle.

The case of Tom Paris is a lesson of how fragile life can be. No one deserves his fate, yet bad things happen. He learned that the responsible party was given a light sentence by a judge because this was her first such offense. Tom resented much that had resulted from a completely preventable accident. With my report, he planned to settle his pending claims, file for retirement benefits, and travel in a friend's R.V. "I'm gonna make lemonade out of lemons, Doc," he pledged.

## The Case of Jimmy Evans: "I didn't see it coming."

For almost three decades, Jimmy Evans was an employee of Roadway Wizards, a highway maintenance company located in Yuba County. He started with the company when he was in his early thirties. He had previously worked in road construction and was familiar with operating dump trucks, road graders, and paving machinery. Roadway had contracts with city and county agencies to maintain the local streets and highways.

In his initial years with the company, Jimmy was the employee who patched cracks and potholes throughout the county. He would do so on his own or as part of a small crew, if the job was more extensive. After winter storms had subsided, there was usually a lot of street repair needed by springtime. One year, damage from an earthquake resulted in the company hiring several temporary workers to fix the roads and overpasses that had been impacted by nature.

Having grown up in a working-class family from Oklahoma, Jimmy was used to hard work and taking direction from others. He fit in with the company and proved to be reliable, which was not always the case for road workers. Some of his co-workers celebrated paydays with quarts of Bud and Subway sandwiches at lunchtime. Some of the workers showed up for work late, if the job was a long distance from the business' equipment storage site. Management rewarded Jimmy's responsible attitude by making him a working foreman with a bump in salary. Periodic incentive bonuses were instituted by a new general manager. If the company finished a big project early or under budget, the crew shared in the profits.

Jimmy's first significant injury came about while he was driving trucks. He hit an unexpected pothole while cruising to a worksite. That incident resulted in the employee consulting with his primary care physician who prescribed physical therapy and pain killers. Several years later, Jimmy filed a claim for cumulative trauma related to the wear and tear of operating heavy equipment, the jarring action of compacters and tamping machines, and muscle sprains due to lifting activities. His company accepted that claim and covered the cost of visits to a chiropractor for periodic adjustments.

On a date in September 2005, Jimmy was operating a street sweeper on a rural highway at 2:30 in the morning. "I thought I got hit by a cement truck. I didn't see it coming," he recalled. Four years after that accident, that's how he described the impact. It was a drunk driver that rear-ended the sweeper which in turn struck a tree off the side of the road. The other driver was lucky. She was driving an old Cadillac sedan with a strong frame. Jimmy was not as lucky. He was trapped in the sweeper with injuries to both legs. It took two hours before he was extracted by firefighters from the wreck. He still recalls a sense of panic when smelling spilled fuel until a firefighter cut the vehicle's electrical power.

Taken to a local trauma center, Jimmy underwent several surgeries to repair fractures and damaged blood vessels in both legs. A lengthy period of recuperation followed. The outcome left him with chronic pain and the need to use of a cane when walking. He was making use of narcotic analgesic, anti-inflammatory, sedative hypnotic, anticonvulsant, and antidepressant medication. Intertwined with his physical pain was numbness in his left leg, which would at times give way, causing him to lose his balance. He had difficulty falling asleep and would wake up due to pain and nightmares. His ability to cope had been severely challenged. Jimmy was routinely irritable and was disinterested in spending time with others.

The accident that ended his working days and resulted in Jimmy obtaining legal counsel. He was receiving Social Security and pension benefits through his union. He had testified at the drunk driver's trial. She went to state prison. Jimmy was living with two adult sons by his second marriage. He was grateful for their continued assistance with shared expenses and household tasks. The accident that ended his career and forced him to use a cane, had also left Jimmy with symptoms and complaints of post-traumatic stress and depression.

This wounded worker's mild cognitive problems with attention and memory were likely due to his physical pain, moodiness, associated low self-esteem, intrusive recollections, and the effects of his drug regimen. Less likely was a traumatic brain injury, so he was not asked to undergo neuropsychological testing. I recommended the continued use of antidepressant medication along with psychological counseling to help Jimmy transition to a retirement that he had not expected. He wanted his case settled and was planning some foreign travel despite his persistent health problems. "Damn it, doc. I got a bucket list that needs some attention," he stated most clearly.

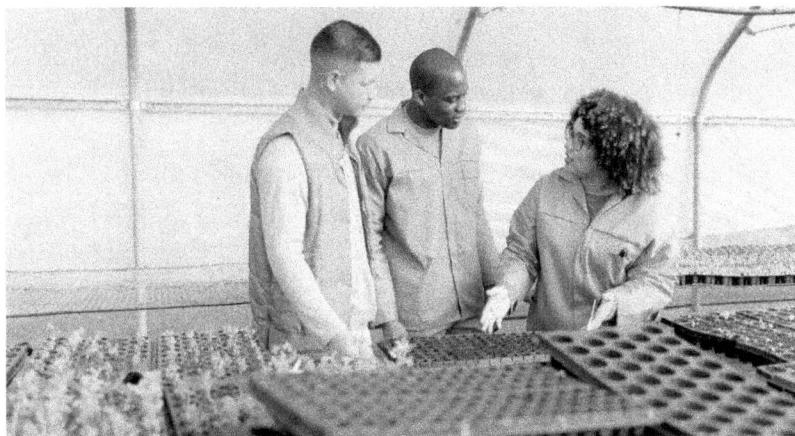

# 11 Landscaping Supervisors: Broken by Terrain

## What Does It Take to Lead a Landscaping Crew?

A working foreman, or supervisor, of a landscaping crew usually has more experience than his co-workers. If fortunate, a $1/hour pay differential may apply along with the title of "Jefe," as in "Boss." These crew chiefs work alongside hardscapers, landscapers, and gardeners.

Landscaping supervisors are the company representatives who deal with clients, oversee the installation and maintenance of projects, train staff, manage irrigation systems, negotiate with vendors, and provide budgetary estimates. These working supervisors are used to working in a broad range of weather conditions, whether on residential properties, in public parks or at commercial spaces.

According to the Occupational Safety and Health Administration (OSHA) the hazards are many for these workers. They include lacerations and amputations; electrical burns; temperature extremes; lifting, carrying, and bending activities; chemical and pesticide exposure; equipment-related accidents; slips, trips and missteps; auditory trauma; and vehicular events.[1]

## The Disturbing Case of Enrico Juarez: An Example of Adaptation

Enrico Juarez was already in charge of a landscaping crew at age twenty-three. He was given the authority to get things done and move on to the next project. It was on a new project where he instructed his crew to lay irrigation piping while he would return a trencher to an equipment rental company. Enrico was moving fast when he "muscled" the equipment into the company pickup. By the end of the workday, the supervisor was satisfied with what he had accomplished, yet his low back was unusually sore.

The next day, after struggling to get out of bed, Enrico could barely move. He reluctantly visited an urgent care center. He was told to rest for two to three days. He did as he was instructed. The pain persisted and an MRI scan demonstrated a disc herniation at L2/3 and a disc bulge at L3/4. Opinions offered by consulting neurosurgeons and orthopedists differed as to what surgery should take place.

Ultimately, Enrico bounced around for years while his case remained unresolved. He opted for a modest invasive procedure compared to the multilevel lumbar fusion that some doctors were willing to perform. This man's long recovery included his becoming addicted to narcotics. When we met, it had been more than ten years since his lifting injury. He was significantly limit-ed. There was a consensus he would never return to activities of heavy lifting and carrying.

I recommended a trial of a nonaddictive antidepressant to address Enrico's chronic pain, sleep disturbance, and depression. He was finally given assistance with his application for Social Security benefits. At a young age, this worker had been injured so badly that he was not going to make a miraculous recovery. Despite a disappointing outcome, Enrico maintained his sobri-ety and was taking steps to become a certified drug counselor. Rather than assume a position of cynicism, he wanted to be of service.

## The Case of a Working Foreman: Guillermo Ortiz Gets Done In

Now at the age of forty, Guillermo Ortiz had been in the U.S. for two dozen years. He spent his childhood on a ranch where he worked from an early age. He was one of eleven children in a family that primarily worked in ranching and farming. He at-tended public schools until age fourteen, when he went to work in fields and orchards picking crops and harvesting fruit. At six-teen, Guillermo came with a brother to Arizona where he was a farm worker for two years before moving to California. He had been with the same building contractor in Santa Clara County for a dozen years. He had such positive feelings about Build It Right Construction that he encouraged a younger brother to be-come a co-worker.

It was on a residential construction site that Guillermo expe-rienced acute low back pain. His job was to set wood forms in place before concrete was poured in constructing sidewalks, re-taining walls, curbs, and driveways. He would cut rebar used to reinforce those features of hardscaping. He was good at his job and became a lead employee for this nonunion crew. Outside of minor cuts and bruises, he had been unscathed by serious injury, until things changed.

Guillermo came to the work with enthusiasm. No one in his family had ever been recruited for a job. In his late 30s, he was offered the position of working foreman, or "El Jefe." Maybe, it sounds better in Spanish. It's a working person's job that has real physical demands, significant stressors, and decent pay. It sounded good to him. What did he know?

As a working foreman, Guillermo had responsibility for the crew's machinery. He was unloading a heavy-duty trencher from the back of a half-ton truck when a ramp collapsed and fell, striking him on the way down. His back pain was too intense for him to continue with his planned work activities. The nurse practitioner at a local urgent care clinic advised he take a few days off. Guillermo described persevering with ongoing pain upon resuming his regular duties. He repeatedly pleaded with clinicians at urgent care to help him. It was a few months after being injured that an MRI scan demonstrated two disc herniations of his lumbosacral spine. A consulting orthopedist recommended removing the discs, fusing three levels of his spine, and inserting hardware in his back.

While Guillermo avoided the complex fusion, he was receiving temporary disability benefits and placed on a panoply of drugs by a "pain management" specialist. He never returned to the landscaping company. Instead, he got a job at a fast-food restaurant and picked up day labor jobs. After hiring an attorney, he was referred for a neurosurgical consultation that recommended the two damaged discs be replaced with synthetic material. The worker became discouraged and confused. He became reliant upon multiple narcotics. The "Candyman," as his doctor was labeled by certain patients, then replaced Guillermo's narcotics with methadone.

I evaluated Guillermo fifteen years after the trencher incident. By then, his marriage had ended. He had spent two years in a clean and sober residence for recovering drug addicts. He had gone to state prison for the use and distribution of illicit pain medication that included fentanyl. In prison, a psychiatrist had placed him on trials of psychotropic drugs.

Guillermo's once-positive future was only a memory. He was destitute and desperate for relief. I recommended he settle his pending claims after far too long. He deserved his care to be overseen by a single physician responsible for all prescription drugs. As prospects for future employment were dim, I advised Guillermo to apply for Social Security benefits. Entering his fifth decade, Guillermo was broken. There was no happy ending for him.

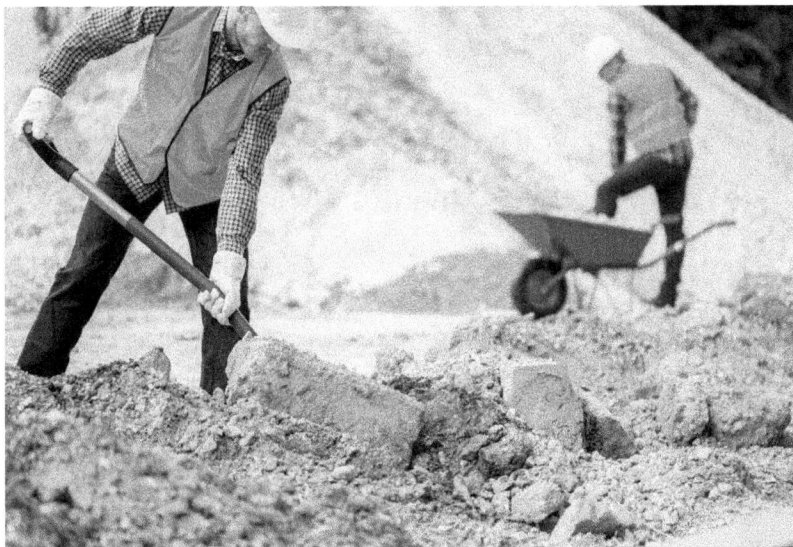

# 12 Construction Helpers: Very Tough Work

*My great-grandfather, Gaetano Iacobucci, came to America in the early twentieth century. His status was that of a "legal alien." Gaetano worked as a laborer on a public works project on Chicago's near-northside. He was part of a crew creating the Lincoln Park Lagoon. He died on the job.*

*His wife and kids never got the details of what caused his on-the-job fatal injury. He was buried in a Catholic cemetery. Guess what his family got? Deported. That's right, as Senore Iacobucci was the only member of his family who could legally be employed, his widow and young children were sent back to Italia. It was my*

*mother and her parents who settled in Chicago several years later.*
*Accidents at construction sites can have serious consequences.*

## How Dangerous Is the Job of Construction Laborer?

According to the U.S. Bureau of Labor Statistics (BLS), falls, slips and trips were the number 1 cause of death for construction laborers in 2020 across the U.S. Those events accounted for 35% of work-related deaths for those employees.[1] Common nonfatal injuries include sprains/strains, fractures, cuts/punctures, and soreness.[2]

## The Case of Frank Villa: Left to Linger

When Frank Villa was part of a crew erecting scaffolding on the site of a new residence in Chowchilla, in south central California, he was a young man in his early twenties. He had been with the stucco company for less than a year. Frank was concentrating on the scaffolding poles when he stepped backwards onto a balcony of the building. Apparently, the flooring had not been completed. He fell through a large space between wooden planks and landed on a concrete slab about ten feet below. He briefly lost consciousness. Thankfully, he had been wearing a protective helmet that absorbed some of the blow to his head. He was taken to a local hospital's E.R., where a brain scan was performed. He was discharged with follow-up to take place through an occupational medicine clinic. There, the physical therapist gave him one treatment session and released him to regular duty.

Frank asked around and was able to get legal representation from a local attorney who handled claims for injured workers. That development led to his coming under the care of a neurologist for persistent headaches as well as neck and low back pain. He remained on a temporary disability status when I saw him.

He was being treated with a mild analgesic, tramadol, and a nonsteroidal anti-inflammatory drug. He had begun taking ESL coursework at a community college.

Frank's personal history found him to have been raised in a working-class family in rural Mexico. He completed his secondary school education and afterwards spent a couple of years working on a ranch with his father. It was after that timeframe that Frank came with a buddy to California. He kept in touch with his family. He had a limited appreciation of the treatment options for his physical injuries. I was being asked to recommend psychiatric care that could get this young man motivated to be productive. There was concern from physicians that some of his neurological complaints made no sense.

Psychological test results seemed to point toward extreme psychopathology consistent with a form of psychosis. This was at odds with Frank's report and behavior when interviewed with the assistance of an interpreter. Rather than recommending treatment with an antipsychotic drug, I assessed much of Frank's clinical presentation to be that of chronic strains/sprains that had been undertreated while colored by a fair degree of symptom exaggeration.

Many of the conservative measures prescribed by the treating neurologist had never been implemented. It seemed that the insurer hoped that Frank would eventually go away. I recommended a nurse case manager get things moving toward the goal of Frank getting back into the workforce. Without this assistance, he might languish while waiting for what was likely a modest case settlement. Oftentimes, addressing the obvious is more productive than going after some rare explanation for what has transpired.

## The Case of Enrique Ortiz: Pain Leads to Pessimism

Now at the age of forty, Enrique Ortiz had been in the U.S. for two dozen years. He spent his childhood on a ranch where he worked from an early age. He was one of eleven children in a family that primarily worked in ranching and farming. He attended public schools until age fourteen, when he went to work in fields and orchards picking crops and harvesting fruit. At the age of sixteen, he came with a brother to Arizona where he was a farm worker for two years before moving to California. He was then employed by the same building contractor in Santa Clara County for a dozen years. He had such positive feelings about Build It Right Construction that he encouraged a younger brother to become a co-worker.

It was on a residential construction site that Enrique experienced acute low back pain. His job was to set wood forms in place before concrete was poured in constructing sidewalks, retaining walls, curbs, and driveways. He would cut rebar used to reinforce those features of hardscaping. He was good at his job and became a lead employee for this non-union crew. Outside of minor cuts and bruises, this worker had been unscathed by serious injury, until things changed.

Enrique was moving a load of rock with the use of a wheelbarrow that got hung up in a small ditch. He pushed through the impediment. Uncharacteristic of Enrique, he asked if he could go home early. He was hurt and his co-workers knew it. When he called in the next day, his supervisor directed this injured worker to a clinic that dealt with occupational injuries. Chiropractic treatment and a series of spinal injections followed. With time, Enrique agreed to undergo surgery to the area of the lumbosacral spine.

While there was some symptomatic improvement, additional consultation led to a variety of medical opinions about how this working man might learn to live with his pain and neurological symptoms of numbness, muscle spasms and weakness. Without much chance for a change in the musculoskeletal problems, this worker would likely remain depressed, worried, irritable, and pessimistic.

## The Case of Armando Aparicio: Lasting Effects of a Hand Injury

Armando Aparicio found work with Gibson Tile and Marble in the community of Tracy, California, after moving with his young wife and kids from Humboldt County. He was used to working with heating and air conditioning systems, until a family member got him more steady employment with Mr. Gibson's company. Armando learned quickly how to install tile floors and marble countertops in restaurants and new homes. He had been with the company for over two years when he injured one of his hands while using a power tool.

Armando was used to cutting tile and stone with electric saws. When doing a remodel, his crew also cut into door jams. That was the task Armando had been assigned by his boss, who removed a safety guard from the saw equipped with a 5-inch cutting blade. "Just be careful," he told Armando. He was careful, yet the saw kicked back and came down on his left hand, which was holding on to a wood surface. One of Armando's co-workers wrapped his injured hand in a clean towel and rushed him to UC Davis Medical Center where doctors performed the first of several surgeries on his injured nerves, bones, and blood vessels.

Armando had badly damaged the ulnar nerve in the affected hand. Doctors harvested donor nerves from both of his legs to be used as grafts in his hand. With time, Armando attempted a return to the tile company, but he now had a claw hand that no longer allowed him to grasp and grip objects easily. He also was too anxious to be able to use power saws. He returned to Humboldt County. Things at home were a challenge as well. Caring for two young children became overwhelming for this man and his young wife. "I've been very moody," he admitted.

Five years after the saw had cut into his hand, Armando's injury claims were expected to be settled. I was asked to weigh in on psychological damages. Multiple previous medical opinions were available to me on the limited function of his left hand. It would never be more than a helper hand. He would not regain fine motor function in the damaged fingers. He was also expected to experience numbness in his legs related to the harvesting of nerves that had been grafted to his hand. Armando had found a customer service position for a tile company in the town where he and his family were now living. He knew a lot about the business, even if he no longer could set tile and stone.

Rather than recommending a potentially habit-forming anti-anxiety drug, I thought that an antidepressant was probably a better choice for Armando's depression and chronic pain. He had been making use of his wife's psychotropic medication, prescribed by a local primary care physician. He was meeting with a counselor to come to terms with his limitations and associated emotional distress when considering his future. Armando started to think of himself as a survivor. This change in his self-image had a therapeutic effect on his state of mind, even though the entire experience had been troubling for him, his spouse, and their two youngsters.

> *Frank Villa fell off unsafe scaffolding and incurred a head injury. Enrique Ortiz injured his back and was given chiropractic treatment, yet he ultimately required surgery. The case of Armando Aparicio is notable for a hand injury, in part, caused by a safety guard that had been removed from an electric saw. What do these injured workers have in common, outside of their job category? All are all immigrants.*

In Chapter 5, the tale of Hector Ruiz includes his unnecessarily receiving a high-voltage electrocution injury. In Chapter 9, Alberto Florio's tale found him requiring emergency neurosurgery for a brain bleed. The sad tale of Guillermo Ortiz in Chapter 11 includes his becoming addicted to pain medication and ending up in prison after he was hurt at work. Like Frank, Enrique, and Armando, all these men were immigrants. A grounds maintenance worker, a cement mason, a member of a landscaping crew, and three construction workers. All were immigrants doing dangerous work that most U.S. citizens would never consider.

I submit these cases are not rarities. The New York Times published an investigative article titled "Fatal Accidents for Immigrants in U.S. Factories."[23] Staffing agencies find immigrants to work manufacturing jobs associated with high fatality rates. In this book, I am telling tales of immigrant workers employed in jobs that may not be in a factory but are highly dangerous for causing life-altering disability and impairment. Whether documented or undocumented, immigrants commonly assume increased safety risks when hired.

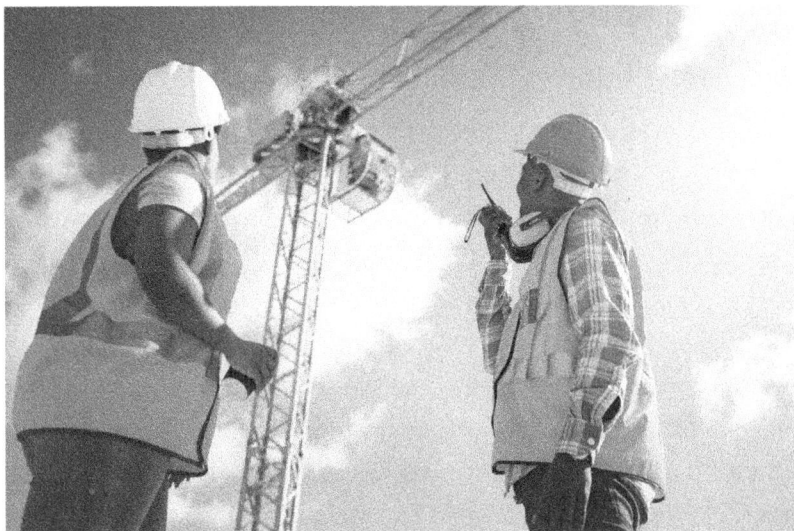

# 13 Crane Operators: Big Machines Are Unforgiving

## What Risks Do Crane Operators Assume?

Crane operators are at risk for electrocution, falling loads, being struck by a swinging crane, being pinned by heavy machinery and loads, and transportation accidents.[1] Once again, big machinery can be unforgiving.

## The Case of George Barnes:
## Take Head Injuries Seriously

George Barnes came to see me in his early 60s, having operated heavy equipment throughout his adult life. At this point, he had been employed by Johnson Construction for thirty years as a crane operator. He'd worked on large-scale projects like BART (Bay Area Rapid Transit) and construction of Highway 280. He took pride in his work and how Johnson had contributed to the San Francisco Bay Area. George was respected by fellow workers and for a time was a job steward for the local branch of the Operating Engineers Union. He wasn't happy at being asked to meet with a psychiatrist.

George was working late on the occasion that brought us together. It was a project at the San Francisco Public Library. While walking on one crane parked next to another, something he'd done many times during his career, he slipped. This time he landed on pavement in the dark and remained unconscious until he awoke in the daylight. Blood stained the concrete where he was resting, and there was a swelling on the side of his head. George was taken by paramedics to San Francisco General where it was determined there was no basis to perform surgery. A neurologist at the hospital referred him on to doctors at a local community hospital for a more extensive work-up.

George found himself struggling with headaches while being told by doctors at the community hospital he had a "mild traumatic head injury." Even though damage to the skull and skin was not impressive, that didn't mean that George's brain was okay. It wasn't. Along with the post-traumatic headaches, he found himself having problems with maintaining his balance, which had never been a problem prior to the head injury. Along with prescription medication for his pain, his neurologist recommended that he take an antidepressant. George resisted, and hence we met up.

Along with the persistent headaches and the balance problem, George had lost much of his sense of taste and smell, signs that the head injury had, in fact, damaged his central nervous system, more than had initially been appreciated. The sensory deficits were annoying, but the balance problem was a potential impediment to George continuing to work on construction sites. He was getting less than optimal care. He wanted to keep working for Johnson, yet to the extent that he could do so had more to do with his perseverance rather than any effective treatment.

This worker's brain injury was largely going unnoticed. It had been several months following his acute injury before our office was asked to get involved. George needed a baseline assessment of his basic cognitive abilities. My colleague, Dr. Eric Morgenthaler, could do so, as he had been trained to conduct neuropsychological testing. This specialized assessment was designed to evaluate areas of concern such as attention, concentration, short-term memory, decision making, judgment, and other areas of executive functioning.

I recommended a form of psychometric testing that goes well beyond giving information about emotions, interpersonal relations, and styles of coping. Such specialized psychological testing is designed to tease out what's going on with persons who have had a documented head injury, toxic exposure that could affect the brain, or a medical condition, whether metabolic or infectious, that would be expected to adversely affect the central nervous system. Our offices have performed these assessments on victims of a one-time injury as in George's case or when a worker has cumulative brain injuries as is well documented for some former National League Football players. (The subject of chronic traumatic encephalopathy was examined in Chapter 25 of *Wounded Workers.*[2])

The test results confirmed that George was having trouble with short-term memory, decision making, and judgment. He would benefit from a program designed for people with a mild traumatic brain injury (TBI). In addition to his follow-up with the neurologist, this injured worker needed to be educated about using cognitive tools such as a daily to-do list. He would benefit from monitoring his progress. Functional improvement could be expected with time and a team approach from additional clinicians with expertise in neurocognitive rehabilitation.

When George returned a few years later, not much had changed. He was still working as a crane operator though he was no longer working overtime or expected to engage in serious physical exertion such as walking on I-beams or performing heavy lifting. He had resisted efforts to see a counselor. "It's not my thing," he demurred.

George continued to take pride in being part of big projects. He liked the income, but he really enjoyed being someone who could be an example and teacher of the next generation of skilled workers. His case was settled with some acknowledgment that he was limited after the fall at work. Not an uncommon outcome if one works long enough around big machines and at heights.

## A Note on Cumulative Injury

Cumulative trauma affects the brain just as it does other body parts. Those cases can often be more complicated than a mild TBI. Modern day football players, especially linemen, are at risk for chronic traumatic encephalopathy (CTE), a type of brain injury brought about by multiple concussions. The brain can be injured by a one-time episode of hypoxia, a reduced level of blood oxygen, or multiple small insults. Think cardiac arrest versus several mini strokes that may go undetected. Workers in certain industries are at risk for exposure to neurotoxins. For example, carbon monoxide is a product of burning various hydrocarbons.

If a singular exposure can be harmful, then repeated, cumulative exposure must be worse. Similarly, closed head injuries in former football players have been found to cause cognitive dysfunction that is distinctly different from cases of elderly patients diagnosed with Parkinson's disease or Alzheimer's dementia. In other chapters, we consider how cumulative physical and psychological trauma can take a toll on first responders. (See Chapters 4 and 17.) Many public safety officers become moody, cynical, and troubled by persistent traumatic memories. This outcome is often a composite of several critical incidents. Bad memories don't just fade away.

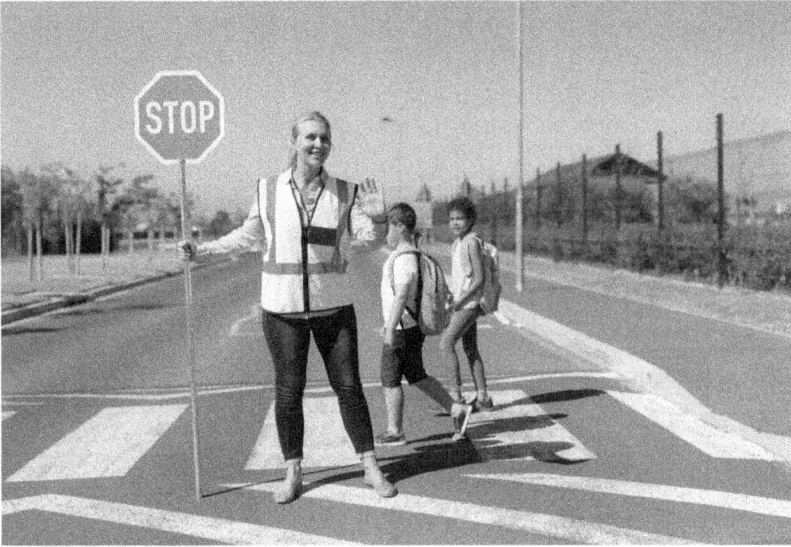

# 14  Crossing Guards: Killed in the Streets

## The Risks to Crossing Guards

Adults who work as crossing guards for school children must be mindful of hazards that go beyond harm to the children. Obvious risks include drivers who are in a hurry and/or distracted. There are also environmental hazards such as cold weather and sun exposure. Crossing guards must be aware of potholes, curbs, and puddles. They should be seen, heard, and carry a whistle. Making eye contact with drivers is a rule worth following. In rural locations, wild animals can come along. Keep in mind the admonition taught to Boy Scouts, "Be Prepared."[1]

## The Sagas of Crossing Guards: Laurie, John, and Rick

Rather than a single vignette, the tales told in this chapter are an amalgam of multiple workers who incurred injury while being out in public, doing their job. Who would have thought being a crossing guard could be so dangerous? Trips and slips, cuts and lacerations, electrical mishaps, heat exposure and freezing rain, avoiding being run over, and facing angry put-downs from passing vehicles. These are the sagas of those folks who walk kids across the street to and from school.

**Laurie Smith** was thrilled to get the part-time job helping where her daughter was starting first grade. Laurie would get to know the school kids and make sure they were safe getting to a small-town elementary school. She completed a training course and was issued a vest with a reflective surface and a whistle to get people's attention. Weeks turned into months, and Laurie became a favorite of the school's pupils. Bright and cheery, that was the reputation she achieved. It was also the reason why some middle schoolers made fun of her. On one occasion, with her back to a group of 6th-grade students, Laurie found herself being pulled off a curb by her long straight blond hair. She ended up on the pavement before she realized an assault was taking place. The school's vice principal happened by and broke up the scuffle. The eleven-year-old assailant was known to administration. The girl had been suspended for spitting on a teacher and for throwing a food tray in the cafeteria. She came from a tough home and hung out with a group known as "The Evil." The crossing guard had a solution. She invited members of The Evil to help walk the special needs kids to class. It worked. No more assaults, no more misbehavior.

**John Gilroy** was a single parent who went to his son's fourth grade teacher with a request to get more involved in the boy's school day. John's workday started early but he was off in the afternoon. Was he interested in taking on crossing guard duties at the end of school? "Sure." So began an afternoon commitment that led to this parent becoming known as "Happy Gilroy." The crossing guard re-upped in the next school year. Everything was going fine until that winter when a snowstorm hit the Sierra foothills while John was safeguarding the kids as they left the school's property. The snow was piling up while the younger children were slipping and sliding. Visibility was becoming minimal. That's when a snowplow turned the corner and struck the guard from behind. John was taken to a local hospital where he underwent a repair of the ACL in his right knee. "Happy Gilroy" became a hero to the school children who two months later presented him with a poster they had painted in their art classes of a man with a big smile standing in a crosswalk.

**Rick Gelotti** was glad to live where his kids grew up with sights of mule deer, raccoons, and elk. The local school needed help from the community, so Rick filled in when he could, hauling trash or putting on a crossing guard vest. In the early fall, in the highlands north of San Francisco, it's the mating season for deer and elk. The rut can go on for weeks. This is when males can be very aggressive. It was an early morning in October when Rick was on duty at the school crosswalk when a bull elk showed up with its mate. Not knowing what to do, the guard tried to clear the wild animals from the area by blowing his whistle. The bull charged, and Rick was left with bruises, a punctured lung, and embarrassment. It could have been much worse. "Next time, I'll stay quiet," he quipped.

The tales I have discussed so far in this chapter have had minor consequences for the workers compared to Tyrone Jones, who was directing traffic as part of a construction crew.

## The Unnerving Case of Tyrone Jones

It was through a vehicular collision report, a prior psychiatric report, state hospital records, and numerous deposition transcripts that I became acquainted with Tyrone Jones. This African American died at age 21 when he was hit by a heavy-duty truck operated by a local water utility district employee.

Most people are unaware that forensic psychiatrists and psychologists are at times called upon to produce autopsy reports. It was the defense attorney for the water district that requested my services. Because the utility district truck had hit Tyrone, killing him and leaving his body in a nearby ditch, his family filed a wrongful death lawsuit.

An investigating officer had generated a detailed report of the accident scene. Tyrone had been hired in a temporary position by the road construction company restriping an intersection on Folsom Boulevard in Davis, California. Tyrone was hired to direct traffic while the work crew completed the task of marking the vehicle and pedestrian lanes on the pavement surface. Tyrone showed up at the worksite on time and had received instruction about his duties from the crew chief. After putting on a reflective vest and hardhat, he set about directing vehicles as they came through the intersection.

It was after a midmorning break that some members of the crew noticed Tyrone engaging in some odd behavior. He stayed apart from the work crew and appeared to be talking to himself. When work resumed, Tyrone was asked by the crew chief if he was all right. He responded with muted laughter. This was followed by the young man putting on a pair of orange utility gloves and walking back toward the intersection. The crew watched as a truck approached. As a crew member directed the vehicle through the area to be restriped, Tyrone pointed at his chest while he stepped off a curb and into the path of the truck.

Two years after his death, Tyrone's case became an unusual injury report for me. The deceased had a history of aberrant behavior that dated back to the age of ten. As a boy, he liked to play with fire. During his middle school years, Tyrone was removed from his mother's custody when it was determined by Family Services, she was an unfit parent. The boy's father was living in another state. Tyrone was made a ward of the state and sent to a special school for boys with behavioral problems. By then, he had taunted other students and spat on a school safety officer.

Tyrone was later reunited with his mother, who had a personal history of substance abuse and minor crimes, including prostitution. She had no idea her son had been identified as an adolescent with special needs. He had already been on trials of antipsychotics, mood stabilizers, antidepressants, and psychostimulants. Mental health professionals had diagnosed him with exhibiting signs of schizophrenia; bipolar disorder; ADHD; an autism spectrum disorder; and a personality disorder with antisocial, borderline, and paranoid features. As he approached adulthood, the future for Tyrone Jones was bleak.

Records from Napa State Hospital in northern California predating Tyrone's death by two or three years tell the story. He was charged with assaulting a police officer, but the court ordered a psychiatric evaluation to determine whether he was competent to stand trial. He was deemed to be a danger to himself and others. The hospitalization was to keep him and the community safe. Six months after admission to the state hospital, Tyrone was discharged to reside in a board and care home, have outpatient treatment through the community mental health system, and be represented by the public defender's office on the assault charge.

Nothing went right. Tyrone was convinced he was the victim of a vengeful government. This was not the first time he had been injured in a traffic accident. The last time, the voice of God had told him he was invincible. He informed his last attorney he could not accept the plea bargain on the assault charge that would find him not guilty by reason of insanity. He could not agree to a label that would follow him forever. He insisted he was not psychotic nor suffering from severe mental illness, when his doctors, nurses, councilors, and aides couldn't even agree upon a diagnosis or treatment plan. He was not wrong that there was never a consensus about Tyrone Jones.

My report did not put the puzzle pieces together. I saw no clear answers about what might have been done differently, so I laid out how Tyrone's life had been lost. One could not hold the truck driver responsible. Who would have predicted the victim's self-destructive behavior? How closely must a company screen prospective employees for a temporary job position? Should Tyrone's unsophisticated family have known what to do with an incorrigible child? Perhaps, the healthcare and legal systems in America have limitations on what can be fixed. The evidence is out in public. Along with the wonder of what humans can achieve, there is also the recognition that some of us cannot care for ourselves. Available public services are often inadequate for those most in need.

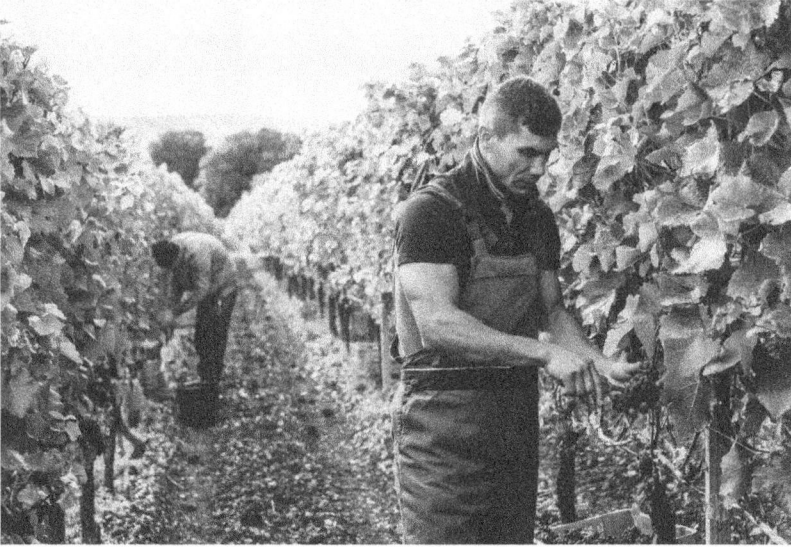

# 15 Farm Workers: Nasty Fields

## Farm Labor Is Heavy Labor

Agricultural workers make use of hands to pick crops, husband animals, and operate equipment. Whether working in fields or in silos, these employees are at risk of injury from objects, big and small. Tractor rollovers and other transportation incidents are commonly a cause for lost-time, i.e., absence from the job, injuries that affect farm workers. Other risks include falls, chemical exposure, sunburns, suffocation, machinery, and livestock.[1] In this chapter, we'll see what happens when a large bovine female contacts a fellow doing his job as a dairy farmer.

## The Case of Manny Fernandez: Hurt While Picking Fruit

He was a man in his mid-sixties and used to manual labor. For the last three years, Manny Fernandez had worked for Sunshine Farms in California's Central Valley on a seasonal basis picking fruit and pruning fruit trees. This was the kind of work he had done his whole life, though he had spent his early years on a ranch in Mexico before immigrating to California for more opportunity. Manny had lived in different areas of that Western state since coming to America.

Manny and his fellow farm workers were picking pears. They did so from a trailer pulled by one of the farm's tractors. When the tractor unexpectedly moved forward, while Manny was standing on the trailer it pulled, he lost his balance. The tractor operator was new to his duties and didn't check with the workers on the trailer before moving to the next group of pear trees. Manny tried to grab hold of a tree limb as he fell off the trailer. He struck his head and back with his coming to rest on the ground. "I started to go dark."

Despite his acute injuries, Manny was a stoic and persevered, performing his expected duties over the next few days. Eventually, his pain was too great, and a fellow farmworker took him to a local hospital, where he underwent a discectomy, disc removal.

## The Case of Benito Juarez: Field Work Hurts

Benito Juarez had been a field worker all his life, dating back to his teenage years. His last job paid him to harvest watermelons in August. It was hot, physically demanding work. Since dropping out of high school forty years ago, Benito was used to what he signed up to do. This was a seasonal job with a farm labor contractor who placed Benito on a crew at a farm near Coalinga, in California's Central Valley. The farm made use of workers who picked the fruit and others who processed the harvest in a large shed. Taking a break from working out in the fields, Benito was selecting fruit for cleaning and boxing for sale.

The worker was attempting to dislodge a large melon that was stuck in the processing machine when the machine operator unexpectedly hit the "on" switch. Benito and his co-workers cried out to shut down the machinery. It was too late. They extracted his mangled left arm from the machine and wrapped it in a clean towel. Paramedics took him to the local hospital where fractures were set with the use of hardware.

Benito had a second surgery and was left with healed fractures of his radius and ulna that did not allow him to do two-handed tasks. The treating surgeon prescribed medication that kept Benito's pain in check. Everyone agreed that this middle-aged man could not return to the duties of an agricultural worker. He admitted to being depressed about his situation yet was thankful for the help and understanding he had from his wife and five adult children.

Through an attorney, his case was settled. Benito was not interested in psychotherapy or a trial of an antidepressant. "I still have one good hand, and my God has a plan for me." He qualified for Social Security benefits and became a deacon in his church where he felt valued.

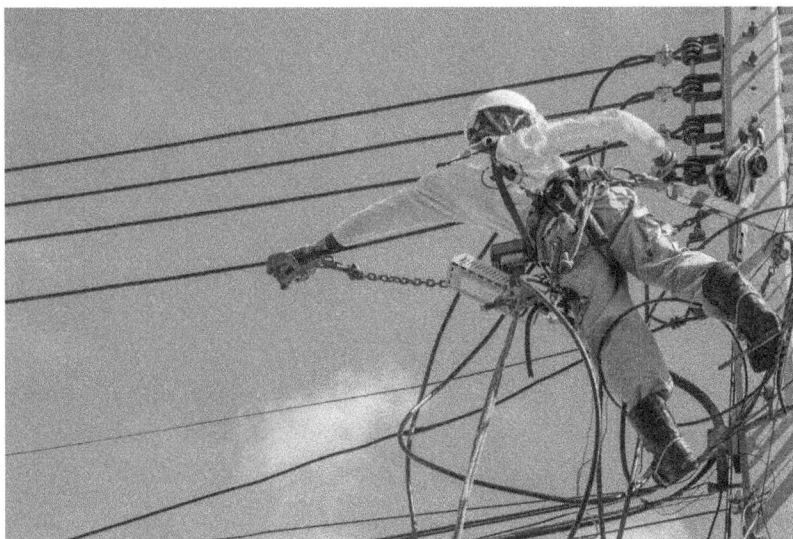

# 16 Power Line Workers: Electrocution

## How Dangerous Are High-Voltage Electrical Lines?

Linemen working for utility companies often work at heights, in underground conditions, in inclement weather, and almost always, around electrical equipment that can burn skin, blow out limbs, and damage internal organs. High-voltage electrical injuries result from contact with lines that carry more than 1,000 volts. Multisystem damage is virtually guaranteed when the human body is subjected to a high-voltage electrocution insult. While such work-related injuries are not common, they have a high mortality rate estimated at 10% to 30%.[1]

Electrical injuries involving high-voltage lines often leave entry and exit wounds. Following acute care for skin burns, follow up can be prolonged. Concern for internal damage requires attention be given for potential cardiac damage.[2]

## The Case of James Craig:
## Shocked, Burned, and Avoidant

James Craig was a 40-year-old lineman for a Bay-area municipality when we met to evaluate his state of mind relative to an industrial incident that had occurred three years earlier. At the time he was injured in the spring of 1999, James was a crew member testing the oil inside electrical transformers. While standing on the ground level, a transformer malfunctioned and sent out an electrical arc that in turn caused the oil to explode. James ended up at a burn center where he spent the next three weeks with second-degree burns to his face, torso, and left arm. He underwent skin grafting to the area of his left elbow. For the next year, he wore a pressure suit while his burned flesh slowly healed. The pain of the burned areas was excruciating.

James reported that loud noises such as fireworks reminded him of the explosion and caused him to feel startled. Along with treatment of his physical injuries, the lineman made use of counseling provided by a psychologist. He found those sessions helpful in dealing with sensitivity about his appearance when venturing out into public. He also came to better understand why he was irritable and blamed his employer for an injury that he considered preventable, yet he alone had to deal with the consequences.

Prior to taking on duties with the city, James had worked for a utility company where he first worked with electrical equipment. "I thought nothing about jumping into a situation where a hot line needed troubleshooting," he recalled. James now finds himself concerned about the potential for reinjury since returning to his lineman duties. He is particularly concerned when working with dated equipment that reminds him of the defective transformer that caused him to be burned over 20% of his body surface.

A recommendation that came out of his psychiatric evaluation was to accommodate this worker's understandable fear of working in underground enclosures with high-voltage equipment. By minimizing his exposure to anxiety-provoking situations where he was expected to service dangerous machinery, James would be less likely to overreact, allowing human error to bring forth more tragedy. His department had enough other assignments for James so that he could be excluded from situations that made him insecure.

## The Case of Robert Rose:
## Convinced He's Been Punished

This skilled worker came to work for a major utility company in his twenties. He had taken some college courses back in his home state of New Mexico. It was after visiting a friend in California's Central Valley that Robert Rose informed his parents that he was smitten by this agricultural paradise. He applied for a job as a painter with the utility company and was hired. He was a crew member painting power towers in the area around Fresno and later throughout the San Francisco Bay area.

Robert especially liked the vast orchards and farmlands in California. He met his future wife when exploring the countryside. She works in the transportation industry. The couple has lived in a rural setting where they have been raising their only son. To remain in the family home, Robert transferred to the company's Tower Division. That resulted in his constructing power towers at locations in the northern half of the state. It was the challenge of a new assignment that led to his being trained for the position of lineman. His crew would perform installation, maintenance, repairs, and decommissioning of electrical lines across the company's vast territory.

Robert considered himself valued until he got seriously injured. While working on a high voltage tower, he lost his balance and fell a short distance. It was not the fall that brought forth his significant injuries. It was his contact with a power line that caused burns with an entry wound on his left hand and exit wounds that involved his legs. He got himself down from the tower, and paramedics transported him to a hospital that had a burn unit. His doctors told him he was lucky. He could easily have suffered permanent cardiac, musculoskeletal, and dermatologic damage. It was only upon hospital discharge that this long-term employee learned that his manager was charging him with negligence. If found responsible for a preventable accident, he could face job termination.

His union stood by Robert. The disciplinary action was resolved with his accepting a warning for recklessness. The employee didn't like the outcome, but he kept his job. No longer trusting his manager, he transferred back to the Painting Division. Continued concern for working with the manager resulted in Robert meeting with a psychologist to discuss his anger and sense of betrayal. He also dealt with lingering anxiety and disturbing dreams related to the electrical burn event. Prior to his accident, Robert had been satisfied with his job. Now, with the support of his wife, he began planning his retirement.

These tales illustrate how direct and indirect effects of a serious physical injury can bring forth a psychological response for the victim. James Craig reacted to his burn injury by being apprehensive and fearful of reinjury. Robert Rose not only had to heal from a blowout injury, but he also had to defend himself from being held at fault. James became less sure of himself, while

Robert could no longer trust management. These are the type of psychological scars that can persist along with the more obvious and visible anatomic defects.

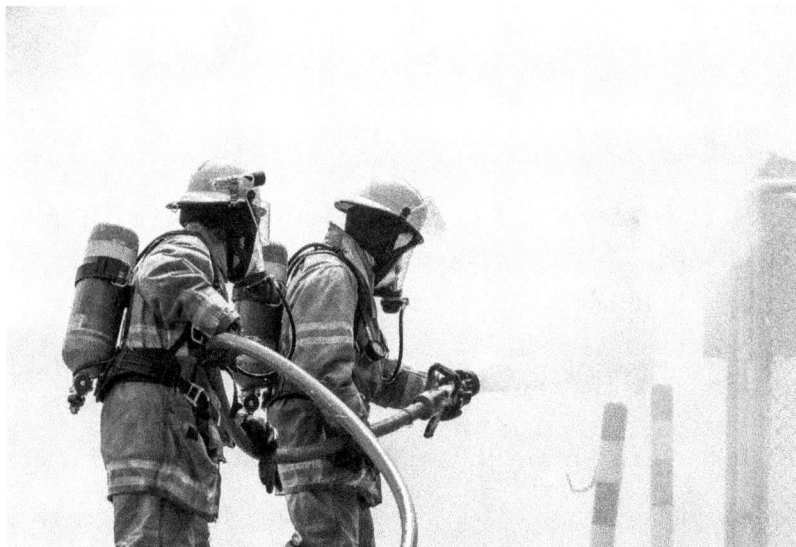

# 17 Firefighters: Hazards Beyond Fires

## What Makes Firefighting Dangerous

Common risks associated with fighting fires include burns, smoke inhalation, crush injuries (often the result of a structural collapse), and heat exhaustion. Long-term exposure puts firefighters at risk of developing chronic illnesses such as asthma, cardiac disease, and cancer. The International Agency for Research on Cancer (IARC) has determined that occupational exposure as a firefighter to be carcinogenic to humans.[1]

Firefighters are commonly exposed to known carcinogens such as asbestos, benzene, formaldehyde, flame retardants, polychlorinated biphenyls (PCBs), and the list goes on. Researchers in the Department of Occupational and Environmental Health Sciences at the University of Washington School of Public Health are studying chemical exposure in career and volunteer firefighters to determine the increased risk for cancer. The goal is to develop preventative measures for these first responders.[2] In addition to physical hazards, firefighters often develop psychological problems that include PTSD and burnout.

## The Case of Captain Jones: Burnout Came About

Captain Jerry Jones, a 15-year veteran firefighter, was referred for a psychiatric evaluation by his labor law attorney and the legal counsel for his employer, a fire department based in the San Francisco Bay area. It was only because of the firefighter being placed on a temporary disability leave for a hand injury that he found himself referred by his treating orthopedist to an employee assistance program (EAP). His EAP counselor recommended a psychiatric consultation, which resulted in the captain being placed on a trial of antidepressant and anxiolytic medication. (Anxiolytic is synonymous with an anti-anxiety drug such as Valium or Xanax.) The firefighter's exposure to numerous scenes of carnage and horror made him a candidate for the West Coast Post-trauma Retreat (WCPR). That five-day program for first responders uses a residential setting staffed by psychologists, clergy, and fellow first responders.

Prior to coming to work for the fire department, Jerry had been a U.S. Marine with combat experience. He never sought out help to deal with life-and-death situations. While he was on a disability leave for his hand injury, his long-suppressed work-related demons surfaced. The suicide of a young child, the death scene of a homeless man, multiple fatal motor vehicle accidents, a toddler's drowning, a woman's dead body partially eaten by a dog, and innumerable critical incidents left the firefighter spent. He presented with a panoply of psychiatric symptoms including intrusive recollections, disturbing dreams, emotional lability, social withdrawal, self-blame, tearfulness, indecision, decreased libido and appetite, and other features of PTSD, depression, and anxiety.

While highly regarded in his department, Jerry no longer saw himself as competent to lead other firefighters. When released to return to work by his hand surgeon, that same physician was highly concerned about his patient's state of mind. The work-related injury claim for the hand was amended to include "injury to the psyche." For some time, the captain had been disengaged from family and friends. He had set aside his interests in camping, hunting, and classic cars. It was while attending the post-trauma retreat that the captain first learned of the concept of "burnout." His peers spoke of a syndrome considered to be a common occupational hazard in firefighters, police officers, emergency medical technicians (EMTs), and other first responders. Reluctantly, the captain filed the paperwork for a disability retirement. He did so because he realized that he no longer had the resilience to confront scenes of human tragedy that had become a regular part of the job.

What is burnout? Why is it common in veteran first responders? Signs of burnout include physical exhaustion, mental fatigue, emotional detachment, cynicism, reduced interest in pleasurable activities, and the list goes on. Burnout is usually the result of chronic work-related stress. Given the cumulative demands associated with the role of a first responder in a busy department, it should not be surprising that cops, firefighters and other employees, whose job it is to respond to emergencies in the community they serve, become victims of burnout. They become wrung out. They often present with symptoms of PTSD, features of an atypical depression marked by irritability and pessimism, a disturbed sleep pattern, and maladaptive efforts of coping such as alcohol and prescription drug abuse.

Programs such as WCPR can help first responders recognize they are suffering from burnout. Recognition can then lead to changes in behavior. Reducing the number of overtime hours can improve one's energy level and mental acuity. Commitment to a regular sleep schedule helps in that regard as well. Finding time to shut off work responsibilities when away from the worksite reduces the likelihood of becoming unidimensional, which can lead to resentment. A good psychologist or counselor can help reinforce healthy actions. Support from friends and family can reinforce positive change that can prolong a career that had been nearing its end. Peer support and departments that recognize the need for some balance regarding work and avocational activities can lead to increased productivity and resilience. Had Captain Jones become involved in activities to offset work-related stress at an earlier point, he may not have experienced burnout that resulted in his early retirement.

## Jane Newcomb's Cancer Results in a Compensable Consequence

In her late 40s, Jane Newcomb was referred for a psychiatric evaluation related to her duties as a firefighter for almost two decades. She had made a career change after having worked for nine years in human resources for two major corporations and a dot.com in downtown San Francisco. She wanted a job that would challenge her physically while giving her the satisfaction of serving her community. When she joined the San Francisco Fire Department, her husband was already a member of the department.

Jane successfully completed training in the department's academy where she was one of two women in a class of forty. This was followed by a one-year probationary period at two firehouses. For a dozen years, she primarily worked out of two firehouses in the Sunset and Glen Park districts of the city. There was also a year when she was assigned to be a dispatcher out of a communications center in the Tenderloin. When I met Jane, she was working as a firefighter at the San Francisco International Airport.

Jane had been involved in numerous scenes of trauma and experienced the loss of fellow firefighters. It was at the memorial service for a firefighter who died in a building fire that Jane "carried his helmet." There were also several of her co-workers who were diagnosed with cancer. She reported that firefighters were "dropping like flies." It was her own diagnosis and treatment for breast cancer that led to our meeting.

In California, there are work-related injuries that are "presumed" to be industrial injuries. These presumptions are based upon public health and labor statistics. This is akin to a pulmonary surgeon assuming his patient's long history of tobacco smoking contributed to that person's lung cancer. Rather than litigate cancer claims, employers, and their insurers, accept that firefighters with sufficient years of service are at high risk of developing cancer through on-the-job exposure. Jane's breast cancer claim was accepted by her employer. What followed was a half-dozen years of medical treatment, periods of temporary disability, and emotional distress.

After undergoing a double mastectomy, Jane was treated by a plastic surgeon who performed reconstructive surgery. Donor tissue from her abdomen was used. That surgery was complicated by a prolonged wound infection requiring drainage and antibiotics. She was left with significant scarring of her chest and abdomen. An expected four-month medical leave turned into a year of suffering. A marriage that had been strained by her husband's alcohol abuse ended in divorce.

Jane's cancer treatment involved surgery and monitoring for signs of recurrence. She did not undergo chemotherapy, immunotherapy, nor radiation treatment. She was grateful for passing the "five-year cancer free mark." Her life had changed in many ways. She could no longer be a blood donor as she had been in the past. She was sensitive about her physical appearance. Back working as a firefighter, she struggled with the job's physical demands. "Working with men, you don't want to be a weak link," she reported.

While Jane had never been treated for depression, she had gotten support from a group for women with cancer. She was keeping up her responsibility for raising two kids while sharing custody with her ex-husband. She had met a new male companion through their shared interest in working out at a gym. Despite keeping an active schedule, Jane was routinely tired, sad, and tearful. Hers was not a case of PTSD but one of an understandable clinical depression.

What good could come of Jane telling me her saga? She wasn't looking forward to having me declare her unfit for duty so she could retire. However, as her claim for an industrial physical injury had been accepted, her depression related to her cancer diagnosis and treatment was also found to be compensable. My report made the case for her depression to qualify as a condition secondary to her physical injury. As such, Jane could now receive psychotherapy for a "compensable consequence psychiatric injury." Her depression was as real as the scarring of her chest and abdomen that was the employer's responsibility. Jane was grateful that she would be referred to a skilled psychologist who worked with cancer survivors. She had a renewed sense of optimism. This was a tale that might end well for both the employer and the employee, given what obstacles had already been overcome.

## The Case of Ed Grainger: An Unnecessary Injury

Ed Grainger worked in a physician's office for some years after graduating from a state university. He enjoyed his time working with patients, but he yearned for work that would be more fulfilling. After consulting his wife, Ed applied to the fire academy in San Francisco. He was a bit older than his academy mates, but he could keep up physically because he had been a competitive athlete through college and later on through community recreation department teams.

Ed was interested in learning the various duties of a firefighter. In his two decades with the department, he worked at all 42 stations. He functions as a firefighter and emergency medical technician (EMT). Ed has competed in the Firefighter Olympics. He has been a peer responder for co-workers who struggle with stress and symptoms of burnout. He has also attended a retreat for first responders dealing with the psychological consequences of the work they do.

Ed's accident occurred one January day when he was working out of a station on the west side of San Francisco. Though he was the most experienced member of the fire engine crew, the crew's lieutenant gave a probationary employee the job of operating the tiller at the rear of the vehicle. After completing a standard training exercise, Ed sat next to that younger co-worker as they drove to a site to refuel. Going around a corner, the tiller operator miscalculated. Preparing for a crash, Ed unbuckled his seatbelt and shouted out directives to correct for the path of the vehicle's back end.

The fire engine hit a large tree. The impact "shredded my seat." While he had avoided a worse outcome, Ed had incurred multiple traumatic injuries. He was accompanied to San Francisco General Hospital by the crew's paramedic. As the county hospital, this hospital is not a place to go for routine outpatient

115

care. It's the clinical site of choice for addressing gunshot wounds and serious motor vehicle accidents.

When I met Ed, it had been almost two years since he was injured. Somehow, a pelvic fracture went undiagnosed. He ended up at another hospital where a surgical team used plates and screws to stabilize his pelvis. The complication of a bowel obstruction required a partial colectomy, or removal of a portion of his intestines. He has also required surgery for injuries to his left knee and low back. Ed takes as little medication as possible. He has recuperated at home with his wife's help.

This man's personal life is not the problem. He and his wife met years ago when selling concessions at sports events. They have three adolescent offspring and have lived in their current residence for two dozen years. He has not returned to work in the fire department, yet he plans to do so when his various injuries are stable and there is an agreement as to what duties he can handle. Ed should be considered a team player who could be a role model for others. As of publication time, the end result remains uncertain.

## The Case of Battalion Chief Edwards: A Very Personal Development

Battalion Chief Edwards came into my office for an evaluation related to his claim for cumulative stress stemming from his twenty-five years as a firefighter. I had read through his records and the cover letter from his attorney. He had completed the standard battery of psychometric tests. He was a neatly attired, middle-aged African American. As he took a seat across from me at my desk, he said, "I think we've met before."

I didn't recognize him. He reminded me of how and when we had first crossed paths. "Oh, yeah. Hit-and-run motorcycle accident, Highway I-80 in Richmond. You were headed to San

Francisco." It all came back, as they say, in a flash. I was in the fast lane when I saw a bit of smoke about a quarter mile ahead. As I slowed down, I could see a biker and his Harley on the pavement. If I moved over to the middle lane, the vehicle behind me would likely hit the victim. Putting on my emergency flashers, I came to a stop without being rear-ended. The drivers to my right stopped as well, blocking all three lanes of a major freeway.

I checked on the victim, who was in a sonorous state after losing his beanie cap when hitting the pavement. Returning to my car's trunk, I got out a blanket and a first aid kit. I came close to being hit by a car driving up the emergency lane to get a better look. Back with the victim, I assessed his injuries, stopped the external bleeding, and covered him up. He had a skull fracture and internal injuries of undetermined severity. I made sure no one moved him, as his spine could be unstable.

I directed a detective who arrived on the scene to get control as cars were stopping on the other side of the freeway to let their kids watch. Then the "bus" arrived. (Fire engines are affectionately known as a form of public transportation, at least in certain firehouses.)

"Are you a physician?" demanded the approaching battalion chief. To which I replied, "Yes, I am. This is my patient. Here's what I know. He's in a deep coma. He likely has cervical spine and internal injuries. His pulse is thready, and his respirations labored. I didn't see the accident. Here's my card. Can I go?"

Four years later, that same battalion chief had walked into my office.

"My attorney says I don't just have physical injuries after doing this job for two dozen years. I have demons. He told me that I was being referred to some shrink named Larsen." In response, the chief reportedly said, "He's a real doctor. He stops at accidents. Of course, I'll speak with him." Our discussion was serious and personal.

The battalion chief was not there because of one accident, rather his "demons" were the result of the exposure to innumerable scenes of horror. I confessed to him that I had prayed for the biker to die. There was not going to be any miracle. The firefighter understood. He proceeded to tell me his tale. His attorney was correct. Battalion Chief Edwards had demons.

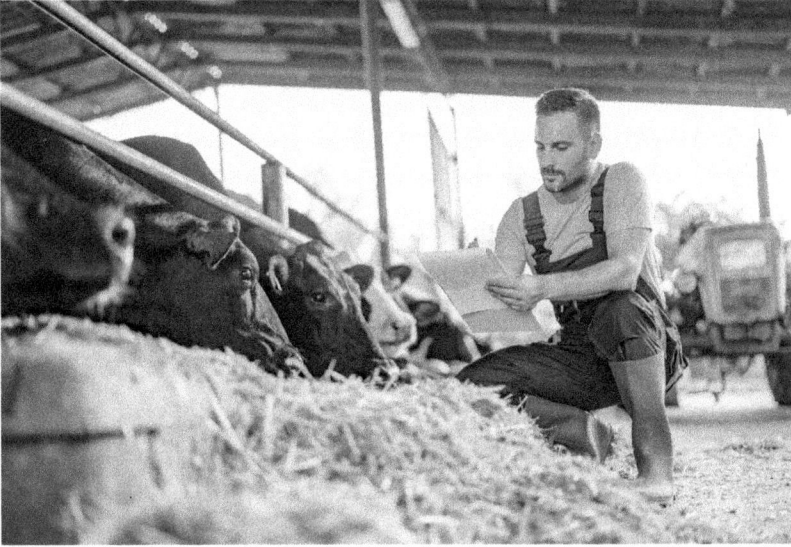

# 18 Farmers and Ranchers: Livestock and Machinery

## How Is Ranching Dangerous?

It goes without saying that working around uncooperative livestock, complex machinery, toxic chemicals, and dangerous pesticides is stressful and puts one at risk for injury and illness. Economic swings in the marketplace add to the uncertainty for ranchers as well. While this segment of our economy has a history of boom and bust, the dangers for ranchers are real.[1]

If things can get worse for humanity because of environmental conditions, that may already be the case for ranching.

Wildfires of biblical proportions raged in Texas in 2024. Ranchers there lost big time. There is a good likelihood there is more to come.[2]

## The Case of a Lifelong Rancher: The Tale of Carlos Quintara

He was a seventy-year-old widower who was dealing with the outcome of an incident at work that had occurred two years before we met. Carlos Quintara had been working on ranches since he was fifteen. He grew up in a small town in rural Mexico where he was raised by his maternal grandmother. He attended public schools in his homeland and did chores on a small family farm. He was sent to live with an uncle in Reedley, California, where he learned about the life of a rancher for the next twenty years on the Pecos Trail Ranch. He went on to split his time between Mexico and California's Central Valley while working at the Lazy J Ranch. Carlos took pride in his understanding of livestock.

Carlos spotted a young calf that was in danger of being crushed by adult cattle in the herd. He took it upon himself to move into the herd so that he could extract the little one before it was injured. Ironically, the calf became spooked and head-butted Carlos in his groin. He experienced acute pain throughout his pelvis. He managed to remove the calf to safety while stumbling along due to pain. He noticed a swelling in his crotch that led co-workers to take him to a local E.R., where he was diagnosed with bruised and inflamed testicles, and treated with anti-inflammatory medication, rest, and ice packs.

While Carlos was told the bruising would recede within days, he experienced persistent scrotal swelling and blood in his urine. He was referred to a urologist who prescribed an antibiotic to prevent a potential urinary tract infection. A neurologist recommended using the anticonvulsant gabapentin to lessen the unrelenting pain. A general surgeon eliminated the possibilities of testicular torsion, an unnatural twisting of the testes, and a ruptured testes due to a penetrating wound. Bottom line, surgery would not make things better.

As he could no longer engage in heavy lifting nor other vigorous activities of ranching, Carlos reluctantly agreed to retire from the strenuous duties he had known for decades. He was receiving Social Security benefits and was ashamed that he could no longer work at tasks that he was good at performing. His account, the medical records, and his psychological testing were consistent with a man struggling with depression, anxious worry, and somatic concerns.

When this man's case was settled, no one celebrated. While his physical impairment prevented him from ranch work, his psychological response to the forced retirement was one of regret, resentment, and frustration. He was clearly depressed about living in chronic pain. He now struggled with feelings of uselessness and hopelessness. He prayed that he might again be a productive contributor for his community.

Carlos Quintara's tale reminds us of how tenuous the existence we have can be relative to an unforeseen event that is life changing.

## The Case of Jimmy McCarthey: Another Livestock-related Injury

He grew up a farmer, like his dad. It was as a young adult that Jimmy McCarthey changed things up by going into the dairy industry. He was hired by Daisy Acres, a family-run dairy farm. Jimmy was raised on a farm that grew crops, primarily corn. He was familiar with tractors and harvesters. His family had some livestock, but that was for 4-H competition and their own consumption. Taking the job on the dairy farm required him to milk, feed, and tend to cows. This included cows in the birthing process.

Jimmy had worked at Daisy Acres for some years when the owner approached him with a business proposition. The family that had owned the farm for a few generations was getting out of the business. There was an option to sell to a commercial entity based in an adjoining state. Alternatively, the owner hoped that Jimmy might be interested in buying the farm if the terms were favorable enough. So, that's what happened.

Jimmy was used to putting in long days. Getting up early, he would check on his herd with particular attention given to injured and pregnant cows. He had a small staff who fed, vaccinated, and cared for the animals daily. While modern machinery was used to milk the cows, the farm maintained some traditions such as having a pasture for grazing.

Jimmy had always been fit. In high school, he competed in wrestling and football. One of his coaches called Jimmy his "farm boy." This was not meant as a compliment. In his fifties, Jimmy was strong and had the physique of someone much younger than he was. He didn't work out at a gym as chores on the farm kept him in good shape. He and his family grew their own vegetables and had fruit trees. He was a content man.

Jimmy watched one of the cows giving birth. He took it upon himself to clean up the calf. His actions were misperceived by the newborn's mother. She headbutted Jimmy who was bent over at the time of impact. The farmer fell onto his right shoulder while employees took steps to separate their boss from the cow and her calf. Jimmy was taken to an urgent care center where he was fitted with a sling after X-rays were taken. Orthopedic follow-up led to an arthroscopic procedure which didn't achieve its expected results. Still in pain after a few months, Jimmy got a second opinion, which resulted in more surgery.

His second surgery was a more extensive procedure where the affected joint was opened and the ligaments explored. The post-op recovery was prolonged. Jimmy was forced to have others do the hands-on work at Daisy Acres. He was not just dealing with his physical limitations, but also, he found himself at odds with the insurance company he'd had for years to cover employee injuries, which included him as well. One additional surgery was proposed to "tweak" the shoulder by removing scar tissue that was expected to "get the grit out of the piston." His workers' comp carrier would not authorize that surgery because an evaluating surgeon had determined it to be experimental. For the first time in his life, Jimmy found himself treated with an antidepressant prescribed by his primary care physician.

I interviewed Jimmy about four years after he was injured. He complained of chronic pain and reduced range of motion in his right shoulder. He was no longer taking pain medication, but he continued to make use of anti-inflammatory and antidepressant drugs. His psychological testing was consistent with sadness, resentment, and somatic preoccupation. While in overall decent shape, the injury, the outcome of treatment, and the process of dealing with the insurer had left Jimmy with lingering hard feelings. It seemed to have aged him.

The farmer was represented by an attorney who was expected to settle the pending claim. Jimmy was continuing to oversee the dairy farm though he had changed insurance companies. He was also considering selling Daisy Acres because his adult offspring had no interest in keeping it. As seen in other tales in this book, this farmer's life was changed by an injury event that impacted his physical health. It also challenged his resolve.

Sometimes there's no happy ending.

## The Misfortune of Manny Chavez:
## A Case of Equipment Failure

Manny Chavez had worked in ranching and farming throughout his adult years. He had worked for at least a decade for each of his two most recent employers, when he was recruited by a farm operation that produced fruit. Manny had been at his duties operating tractors for only a couple weeks when he was crushed.

The tractor operator had been cultivating the land in preparation for a new season. It was on a December morning when he was spraying fruit trees on the large property where Manny worked outside of Fresno. He intended to fill up the spray tanks that the tractor pulled around the property. There was no hand brake on the tractor, but he assumed it was in a safe idling position. As Manny tried to disembark, he felt the machinery rolling. In his attempt to jump free, his clothing got caught. He ended up on the ground while the tractor and the spray cart rolled over him.

It took some time before other farm employees came to check on Manny. When paramedics arrived, there was a debate as to how the accident victim should best be transported given his extensive injuries. At a community hospital, he underwent surgery related to fractures of both femurs. He was later readmitted to undergo surgical removal of hardware. In addition to his orthopedic issues, he has been offered counseling from a psychologist with a focus on his dreams and memories of the injury event.

I met Manny more than two years after the date of injury. He was taking pain medication for complaints of right hip and left leg pain. He also was taking an anti-anxiety drug because he frequently felt nervous. Evaluation of his persistent physical symptoms and complaints gave little hope this man in his fifties could resume farming or ranching. Recommendations were made for treatment with an antidepressant that could help with both chronic pain and depression. Manny could also benefit from assistance with his application for Social Security benefits. He was thankful for the assistance of three adult offspring who routinely came by his home of several years.

*I grew up in what had previously been a farming community some miles southwest of Chicago. When my family moved to the town of Orland Park, I was about to begin the first grade at the local elementary school. The official population was listed at just over 700. I made new friends, some of whom lived on farms. There was a one-room public library in town. There was no pizza parlor. My brother and I either walked or rode our bikes to school. By the time we started high school, things had changed. We took a bus to and from school. There were also classmates from less rural communities.*

*Over decades, most of the family-owned farms have sold. Chain restaurants, shopping malls, and housing developments have replaced what had been farmland. For the dairy farmers and agricultural farms that grew corn and other crops, the work was hard, the equipment became expensive, the kids wanted a different life, and the land became too valuable. The population of my once small town is well over 100,000. Things change. Some consider that change to be progress.*

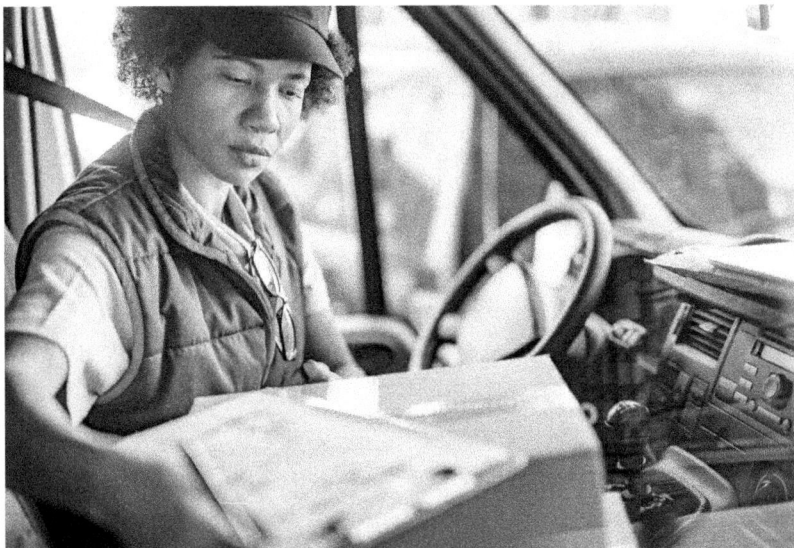

# 19  Delivery Drivers: Crashes Are Common

## Crashes: The Usual Risk

Delivery drivers confront numerous hazards in getting packages to their intended delivery point. This includes collisions, pedestrian traffic, loading activities, carrying packages, trips, and falls.[1] There are also confrontations with members of the community.

For the workers who deliver our goods, whether to businesses or to our homes, motor vehicle accidents often cause injury, the need for emergency medical services, and even death. Whether union drivers or independent contractors, these truckers are at increased risk for hitting a roadside hazard, leaving the roadway due to weather conditions, being t-boned in an intersection, or ending up in a multi-vehicle crash than people who do not drive as a key work activity.

Aside from vehicular accidents, delivery drivers experience lifting injuries, are injured by heavy equipment, become exposed to chemicals and biohazards, and can end up in confrontations with customers as well as co-workers. These confrontations can turn violent, especially when workers are confronted with firearms. In this chapter, we see the aftereffects of America's gun violence epidemic on three employees and on a workplace that will never be the same.

## The Cases of a Shipping Hub Mass Shooting

It was the start of a normal workday at this international corporation's shipping center in San Francisco. The drivers gathered around for their morning report while the last packages were being loaded onto their package trucks. Nothing seemed out of the ordinary until the chitchat was interrupted by the sound of gunfire.

**Lin Chiu** had been a package truck driver for the company for a few years when he heard a ruckus and loud bangs at a distance across the trucking center. He recalls moving toward frightened drivers and then turning away only to find himself shot in his right leg. Upon exiting the building, to find safety, he saw co-worker Sam Wee armed with a handgun. Another driver was wounded and lying on the pavement. Returning inside, Lin took shelter in an office. Two San Francisco Police Department (SFPD) officers found him there and brought him outside where pressure was applied to his leg wound. From there, he was taken by ambulance to San Francisco General, a county hospital and trauma center. A determination was made that a through-and-through path of the bullet had caused no fracture nor any damage to major blood vessels.

Lin was discharged that day when his adult daughter and a cousin took him home. At the hospital, he learned that other drivers had also been shot. Lin came under the care of an internist, Dr. Lo, and a psychologist, Dr. Lee, both of whom were fluent in Cantonese, as was Lin. Fifteen months later, he returned to modified duties that limited the weight he should lift. Lin returned to regular driver duties about two years after the mass shooting.

Like other drivers who were present during the shooting incident, Lin had been provided with counseling, in addition to the attention given to his physical injury.

When I evaluated Lin, four years after the mass shooting, he was still suffering from post-traumatic stress and depressive symptoms. The driver's case was settled with an award for his persistent physical and mental symptoms, such as recurrent recollections and fear for his safety. While he was expected to reduce the frequency of psychotherapy and discontinue such in the next few years, he was deemed to be capable of continuing to work at the site where the shooting had occurred.

**John Lo** had been with the shipping company for a decade working in a warehouse and later as a loader. He became aware that something was terribly wrong as co-workers ran by him the morning of the mass shooting. "Someone yelled, 'Shooter, shooter, run.' So, I did." Outside the shipping center, he heard gunshots and saw Mr. Wee holding a gun. Another driver was motionless on the asphalt. John followed other employees who put some distance between themselves and the shipping center. When returning to the worksite that morning, he was directed to a local church where SFPD patrol officers and detectives interviewed him. He learned that he worked regularly with two drivers who had been shot and killed by their fellow driver, Mr. Wee.

John ended up on a leave of absence and referred by his employer to a psychologist "who just wanted to know when I'd be up for going back to work." Meanwhile, John found himself preoccupied with the deaths of fellow employees. Of the four who died that day, he knew two victims and the shooter. It was after obtaining legal counsel, upon the advice of another employee, that John went to see a second psychotherapist, who helped him return to work. It took several months for him to do so only to find another worker confront him by saying, "Why do you think you needed time off? You didn't get shot." After that, his therapist placed him on a temporary disability status again. He resumed his job duties a few months later. By then, he had ended all treatment.

Three years after the shootings, I met with John. He reported that he was regularly startled by loud noises. When away from work, he avoided spending time with his wife and young child. While he could keep working, additional psychotherapy and a trial of an antidepressant were recommended to address chronic PTSD and a major depression. I expected to reevaluate things on a future occasion for this employee, who had become victimized.

**Ed Yung** was in the circle for the morning report when a loud pop caused him to turn around. "There he was with the gun in his hand," Ed recalled. Ed jumped under a vehicle and remained still. More shots were fired. People ran off. Some time elapsed during which things got very quiet. Hoping it was safe, Ed got out from under the vehicle. The only employees he saw were two drivers lying in pools of blood. He could see there was nothing he could do for them. He heard someone cry out, "He's coming back." So, Ed returned to his hiding place. This cry that the shooter was coming back was a false alarm. This time when he got out from hiding, he saw his female manager, who oversaw the morning report, standing near the two dead drivers, unable to say anything.

Dozens of employees fled the building from the ground level *en masse*. Word got out that a collection point had been established at a local church. Later in the afternoon, Ed was interviewed by a police officer. He drove himself home. The next day he went by work, which he described as being in disarray with boxes strewn about. After reporting to his manager that he had a bruised elbow, Ed was referred to an occupational medicine clinic at the San Francisco Giants ballpark. He came under the care of a neurologist and a psychologist. It took two years before he was ready to resume his driving duties.

Unlike Lin and John, who had spent their childhood in China, Ed had grown up in Vietnam before immigrating to America. However, like those co-workers, he had never made use of mental health services before the mass shooting. Along with treatment for orthopedic problems involving the elbow and shoulder that had come forth because of his hiding out during the incident, Ed learned that he was having difficulty letting go of his fears, mistrust, disturbed sleep, and moodiness. He was returning to driver duties while continuing to have orthopedic and psychological follow-up. I recommended a trial of an antidepressant to address complaints of depression, difficulty falling asleep, and chronic pain. That was four years after the shootings. As I had with others, I told Ed that what he was experiencing was "normal, but not healthy."

**Janet Grant** had been with the shipping company for a half-dozen years when she heard loud popping sounds and the screams of fellow drivers on that June morning. Janet had been organizing packages for delivery rather than be part of the morning meeting for drivers assigned to the Presidio Center. She called out to a nearby male co-worker, who joined her in the delivery truck. The two employees proceeded to barricade themselves inside the vehicle. The gunshots and shrieks of terror seemed to go on interminably. Janet called 911 and remained on her cell phone with a dispatcher. Quiet followed until members of an SFPD SWAT team ordered the occupants of her truck to show themselves. Janet was "frisked" and then escorted to a nearby church for questioning. "I think they were detectives," she explained The employees returned to the worksite to gather their belongings hours later. "There was all so much blood on the floor."

Janet later learned that four employees had been shot and killed that day. This included a driver who had clocked out and was leaving the worksite. Before reaching the car where his wife was waiting, the off-duty employee was gunned down. He was the driver who had encouraged Janet to apply to the company years before.

Nothing seemed to make sense to Janet in the weeks that followed the workplace mass shooting. She had been seeing a counselor before this tragedy, termed a critical incident by investigators, occurred. Those sessions continued while she was placed on a disability leave. A consulting psychiatrist recommended trials of antidepressant and anti-anxiety drugs. Janet had been abstinent from alcohol for a few years before the mass shooting. She preferred to take no psychiatric medication while she went to counseling, had contact with her psychiatrist, and attended A.A. meetings. She told me when unable to sleep, she'd make use of cannabis.

Six months after the shooting incident occurred, Janet attempted a return to her driver duties, having been released to do so by her treating doctor. That psychiatrist sent in a final report, ending treatment. This was despite evidence that Janet was still having symptoms of anxiety, fearfulness, and avoidant behavior triggered by loud noises and news accounts of other unrelated shootings.

When I met Janet, it was at the request of her workers' comp attorney. She was also involved in civil litigation, as one of several plaintiffs, suing the security company for their worksite. The gunman had smuggled two semi-automatic weapons into the shipping hub on the date those firearms ended four lives and changed the lives of so many others. Janet had been off work with a reported physical injury, which was not contested. She made clear her disinterest in resuming her driving duties. She had begun a dog-walking service. I made recommendations for treatment, job retraining, and case settlement. Janet was lost to follow-up.

After meeting with thirteen of the victims of the mass shooting at the shipping hub, I informed the employer, their attorneys, and the insurer that I thought it best that I not meet with any more of these employees who gave a variation on a theme of senseless gun violence.

Was Mr. Wee mentally ill? Was he so angry, for whatever reason, that he opted to kill some people he didn't know and end his life. An unexpected twist to this saga involves Chapter Four of this book. The detective who investigated the shipping hub mass shooting is portrayed in that account of "To Serve and Protect." A tough cop meets up with a tough shrink, perhaps only to acknowledge that we all have our limits in confronting human suffering.

Gun violence in America has reached epidemic proportions. On average, mass shootings take place every day. In *Wounded Workers*, Chapter Four, titled, "We Have a Problem with Guns," gun violence is addressed as a public health issue.[2] As a physician who sees the casualties, I must ask, "When is enough, enough?" While the U.S. has more firearms than citizens, most Americans don't own a gun, much less an AR-15–style weapon. Residents of civilized countries across the globe get by without the type of firearms that are readily available to Americans. How will history judge us on this contentious issue?

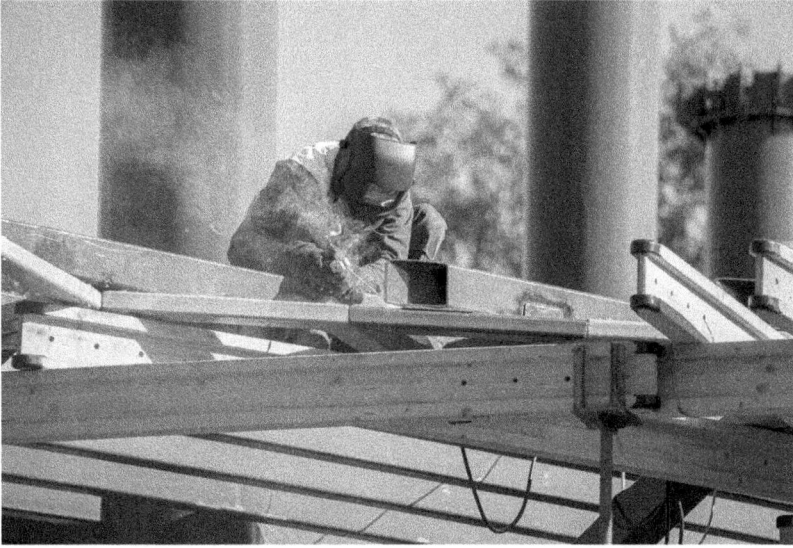

# 20 Ironworkers: Heights and Other Hazards

## How Do Ironworkers Get Hurt?

Aside from falls from heights, ironworkers commonly are subjected to cuts and lacerations, amputations, crush injuries, being struck by objects, electrocution, and even burns. Hazards typical of construction sites are elements of what iron workers confront daily. A high fatality rate involves falls, being struck by steel beams, crush injuries from collapsing concrete, and contact with power tools and electrical lines.[1]

## The Case of Tom Smith: Determined to Live On

Tom Smith grew up in a town of 2,500 in California's Central Valley. This region is known for farming fruits and vegetables as well as large-scale vineyards. Tom's father was the owner and operator of Smith Iron Works. Tom was the younger of two children who were raised in a middle-class household. Family activities during his youth involved camping, boating, and outings to parks and the local zoo. Tom had acceptable performance through high school. He married his high school sweetheart. He also took some drafting coursework before going to work in his father's company.

Tom was an ironworker employed by his father for six years, after which time the business was sold. With that development, he was hired by a larger company in a union job position. Valley Steel was responsible for constructing steel framing for high-rise commercial buildings in central and northern California. Tom came to be seen as a dependable, skilled employee who needed little supervision. He was routinely asked to prefabricate steel structures that were intended for projects at other locations. He did that work for fifteen years until a singular event ended his career in construction.

Tom was tack welding metal framing as he had done hundreds of times before. Once his job was complete, a welder would finish off the welding, thus making the structure more solid. Tom was finishing off a job when a spark from the torch landed on his flannel shirt. The protective apron he was wearing did not completely shield him from the hazard his clothing ignited. He had the presence of mind to hit the floor and roll about. Even with the assistance of a co-worker, there was some difficulty getting the apron and fiery garments off. Tom recalls his acute pain as worse than he could have imagined. Paramedics arrived and decided to medevac the ironworker to a major medical center with a dedicated burn unit.

At the burn unit, the medical team assessed the extent and severity of Tom's burns. They treated him with intravenous fluids to mitigate his risk of entering a state of shock. They administered narcotic analgesics to help with the pain. They applied dressings and antibiotic ointment to his superficial wounds. Within days of his admission, once he was stable, a series of skin graft procedures began to remove seriously damaged tissue in the areas of his right arm, right shoulder, and much of his back. Donor skin was taken from areas on his legs. Following these initial procedures, Tom was transported by ambulance to his home, where specialized home-care services took place. His lengthy period of recuperation included many months of physical therapy, which he described as "horribly painful."

Tom got through the first year following the work-related accident without blaming himself or his employer. As his physical pain lessened, he still found himself moody, sensitive about his scared physical appearance, and experiencing dreams and flashbacks about catching on fire. His attorney referred him to a psychologist whom he saw for a few months when getting back out into the community. A major issue for this worker was the firm recommendation by all his doctors that Tom should not return to iron working. His sensitivity to heat was too great for him to resume duties that could further damage the skin covering much of his torso. With some reservations, he met with a vocational counselor to begin the process of retraining.

Nearly four years after Tom had been burned, he had an appointment with me. Tom put forth relevant information in a logical manner, without hyperbole, though he occasionally used some colorful language to describe his burn wound pain. Tom had completed an 18-month course of study to become a pharmacy technician. He was working as an apprentice in a pharmacy while in his mid-forties. While his chronic pain was under control, he avoided sun and heat exposure.

Tom had ended counseling as he did not wish to relive "the day I caught fire." News segments about fires triggered traumatic recollections. As a man who had always kept in shape, he described being sensitive about his appearance. After frightening a young boy who saw him with his shirt off, Tom made a conscious effort not to have further occurrences. "I look like some kind of freak to strangers," he stated. Unrelated to his injuries, his marriage ended. He had raised three children who remained in his custody after the divorce. Despite all that he had gone through with his career-ending injury, Tom had a sense of pride in his resilience and ability to adapt. He expected to settle his pending claims based upon the evidence of persistent scar tissue, pain, post-traumatic symptoms, and mild depression. "My parents didn't raise no wimps."

## The Case of Juan Andre: A Trip in Time

Juan Andre was a proud man. He came from a rural, working-class family in Mexico with a minimal amount of formal education. He was a teenager when he came to California with a paternal uncle. For a few years, he was a farm worker. He had friends who worked in the construction trades. The pay was better, and the work seemed to be steadier. California was growing, and there was a need for housing and commercial space. So, on a visit to the San Francisco Bay area, Juan found a contractor who needed a helper/laborer. He was a construction laborer for some years until he became an apprentice in the local ironworkers' union.

Over time, Juan proved himself to the owner of Gilroy Reinforcements. This was a company that put steel reinforcements in bridges, overpasses, and high-rise structures. Juan could walk the walk with any of his fellow ironworkers, at whatever height and under whatever adverse conditions.

138

In the summer of 1995, the tip of Juan's steel-toed work boot caught on some scrap metal lying on the ground at the worksite that changed his life. This single event resulted in significant damage to his lower back. After he agreed to undergo removal of an intervertebral disc and a fusion of the adjoining vertebrae, he was not relieved of his pain, nor was he better able to carry rebar at a jobsite. What do you do with plenty of experience in building structures while having no trade certification, yet being at increased risk for future injury? Pray.

We met a half dozen years after Juan had tripped at the worksite. He was now in his late 40s. His discouragement was recognized by the doctors and nurses where he was followed for the effects of his work-related injury. After agreeing to a fusion of the L4 and L5 vertebrae, doctors told Juan another disc needed to be removed. That surgery left his spine even less flexible. On a good day, Juan's pain had lessened. Was he any more capable of resuming his ironworker duties? No.

To make this man's situation more complex, he was recognized as having severe coronary artery disease. His spine surgeon was wary of removing a bone graft stimulator intended to help fuse his low back. The medication regimen included a narcotic analgesic, an anti-inflammatory drug, and a tricyclic antidepressant that had not been a first-line antidepressant for a couple of decades. Neither Juan nor his surgeon wanted to confront the treating psychologist on her vague treatment recommendations

I recommended a trial of a first-line antidepressant. At 48 years old, was it too late for this man to find an alternative career path? If so, Juan needed assistance in pursuing disability and rehabilitation benefits for a worker at the end of his career as a man of steel.

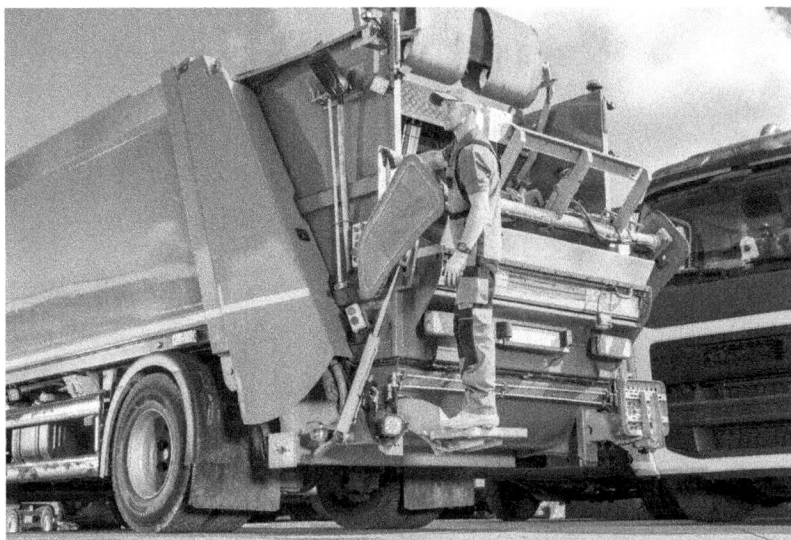

# 21 Refuse and Recyclable Collectors: Accidents Are Frequent

## Whether You Call It Garbage or Refuse, the Work Is Risky

According to data from the U.S. Department of Labor's Bureau of Labor Statistics, employees who collect trash and recyclable materials had the seventh-deadliest occupation in 2021 across America. Approximately 75% of workers in this job category incurred some form of industrial injury that year.[1] Refuse collectors are at risk of being struck by vehicles or injured while standing on a riding step. These types of accidents are the leading cause of death for these employees.[2] Aside from vehicle-related injury, this category of employee is at risk for back problems and hernias related to lifting and carrying activities; sprains and strains due to falls; cuts and lacerations; and toxic exposure. It's dirty, hazardous duty.

## The Case of Vince Giamatti: Damaged by Repetitive Trauma

Vince Giamatti grew up in a working-class Italian American family in a suburb of San Francisco. His dad was a car mechanic. His mom was a housewife who drank too much. Vince was the youngest of three kids. His parents divorced before he started school. Vince was raised by his dad while his older brother and sister stayed with their mother. He struggled in school. He had repeated a grade in middle school. He liked going fishing and bowling with his dad. At fifteen, he ended up briefly in Juvie Hall related to his involvement in a physical fight at his high school. In the eleventh grade, Vince dropped out because he was good with his hands and wanted to make some money.

Throughout his late teens and early twenties, Vince worked at "drivin' jobs." He became self-employed moving and hauling furniture, equipment, and trash. He was a one-man crew who operated a dump truck that he bought with cash. On big projects he would get help from a buddy, but usually he worked alone. He was known in the community by employees of retail shops, movers, the local dumpsite, and a couple garbage companies. That led to his being offered a union garbageman job with Southside Scavengers when he was thirty. Vince would spend the next twenty-five years working for Southside in whatever the company needed him to do.

I was asked to consult with Vince after a series of physical injuries had left him beat up, used up, and broken. Industrial injuries had required surgery to his right hand, right shoulder, and right knee. Vince returned to work after these separate injuries and surgeries. A puncture wound resulted in a right elbow infection that was treated by incision and drainage. Vince was still on antibiotics when he resumed duties for the waste management company.

A couple of years before his appointment with me, this hard-working man found himself having bouts of acute pain in his right groin. After consulting with a few different physicians, it was determined that chronic lifting activity had caused a low back sprain and an inguinal hernia. The sprain was treated with an injection. The hernia would require surgery. Vince was off work and languishing while awaiting a follow-up appointment with his general surgeon. This last injury would prove to be one too many. Delay in the invasive procedure being performed led to the hernia becoming so large that nerve damage occurred in the groin region. To make things worse, a post-operative infection required intravenous antibiotics.

During my interview with Vince, he complained of near-constant pain in his low back, as well as numbness in his right leg and throughout his groin. He moved about slowly and deliberately in our offices. Erectile dysfunction, which followed the hernia repair, had not responded to "that drug that makes your dick hard." Vince had come under the care of a pain management doctor who had his patient take narcotic analgesic, anticonvulsant, muscle relaxant, and antidepressant medication for a recognized chronic pain syndrome. Along with his pain, this middle-aged, injured worker was dejected, frustrated, and miserable.

It was clear that Vine was not a candidate for returning to any regular employment. He was receiving long-term disability benefits, yet his application for Social Security disability benefits had been denied. Psychometric testing was indicative of a person who was dealing with anger, depression, anxiety, and worry over his health and future. He and his wife of thirty years had

143

relocated to a more affordable community. All his life he had been a fisherman and had enjoyed going to car shows. Now, he no longer felt able to go fishing, and he hadn't gone to a car show recently. "I'm just not good for much of anything, Doc," he lamented.

My report couldn't fix Vince, but it did help him to get his deserved disability benefits. He also deserved a consultation with a urologist to address his sexual dysfunction, which was a source of shame for Vince. This man's case is an example of how repetitive physical stress and injury take a toll. Sometimes, there is no miracle from modern medicine that can undo the damage done.


## The Case of Antonio Vera: Please, God, Forgive Me

This is the tale of a man who was thankful for having a job that covered the expenses for his family. He came on board more than twenty years ago when the company primarily handled waste, recyclables, and potential toxins in and around San Francisco, the city he had lived in his entire lifetime. He initially drove large trucks to a dump site outside of that city. He continued in his union job when assigned to a crew of three, where he drove a trash truck while his two co-workers emptied trash and recyclables into their respective bins in that vehicle. The routes changed over the years, but the work was steady.

Ten years into his employment with San Fran Trash, Antonio injured his low back. He learned to live with intermittent discomfort. He never required surgery. He avoided heavy lifting as recommended by his treating doctor.

Three years before his consultation with me, a tragic event landed Antonio in outpatient treatment for depression and PTSD. While driving his garbage truck, Antonio collided with and ran over a young bicyclist. Antonio heard his crew yelling for him to stop. When he did, he saw the bike rider and his bike lying in an intersection behind the truck. While Antonio was making a right turn, the teenager tried to get past the vehicle but miscalculated. Hitting the truck, the bike and its rider fell to the pavement. The truck's rear tires ran over the boy and his bike before Antonio knew the boy was there and stopped. The boy died of his injuries.

Antonio was taken by police for drug testing and an investigation began during which time Antonio was placed on a leave of absence. He was not found to be criminally responsible for the death. While away from his job duties, the driver was referred for counseling and treatment with a first-line antidepressant. Years earlier, Antonio, while going through a divorce, had been treated for depression. Now he was going through another episode of depression that included post-traumatic recollections of the accident scene.

When Antonio resumed his work for the company, he was welcomed back by dozens of his co-workers. That helped.

He also had a letter from the victim's mother waiting for him in the employee locker room. That didn't help.

Antonio and the employer became defendants in a wrongful death lawsuit brought by the bicyclist's family. While provided with legal services, Antonio was troubled by having his deposition taken. The company settled that civil case before it went to trial. By then, Antonio had been back at work driving a debris box truck to the dumpsite for more than a year.

From all accounts, Antonio was a decent fellow who had been raised as the eldest child of Mexican immigrant parents. While his mom worked for a candy company, once all three kids were in public schools, his father worked for S.F. Trash. That parent was responsible for Antonio being hired years later. While a product of public schools, Antonio went to a local Catholic church with his family on Sundays during his youth. He played on competitive soccer teams until he began full-time work for a construction firm, which predated his time with the trash company. This came about after he graduated from high school and had married as a young man.

Antonio divorced after ten years of marriage. He became the custodial parent for his two children. It was during the breakup of his marriage that he was treated for depression. A few years later, he was introduced to a woman by his younger sister. After dating for a couple years, they agreed to marry. His fiancée had no children of her own yet enjoyed time with his kids. Plans for a wedding were taking place while the bride-to-be moved in with Antonio and the children.

Antonio had stopped meeting with his psychologist when his consultation with me took place. It seemed prudent for him to continue taking a low dose of the antidepressant and attending occasional A.A. meetings while he maintained his sobriety. He was continuing to work for the trash company, yet he looked forward to a time when he could retire as his father had from the company. For Antonio, his faith had made a difference in forgiving himself for the bike rider's death.

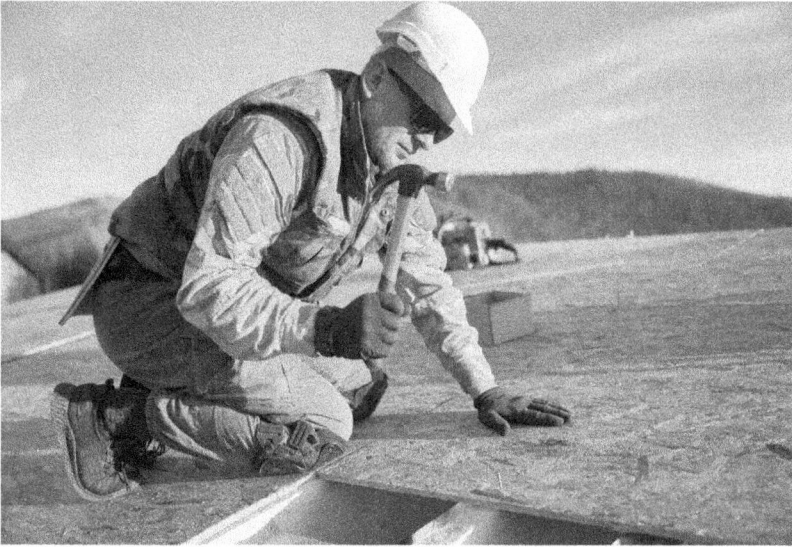

# 22 Roofing: Numerous Hazards

*As a young man living in Miami, I was asked if I wanted to make some extra money working a weekend job. My roommate Ben was a fellow about my age who was part of a roofing crew. His crew was installing a new roof on a home some distance from where we lived. An extra pair of hands were needed to get the job done. As I could use the cash and had no other plans, the roofing assignment became an opportunity and perhaps an adventure.*

*On a Saturday, I sat on the back end of Ben's motorcycle as he drove us on an early morning excursion to the worksite, some fifty miles from our rental property. I became the low man on the totem pole of the roofing crew. This meant I got to carry hod, so to speak. The worksite was a one-story ranch-style house. It was very much a low-tech job. There were four of us tasked with removing the existing composite shingle roof and replacing it with a new one of the same type.*

*While the other guys tore off the old and tossed the materials down to earth, I moved the junk to a heap for disposal. I did so while being mindful not to get hit by falling debris. Old shingles, tar paper, and chunks of wood with protruding nails rained down throughout the morning hours as the existing, worn-out roof was deconstructed. The conditions were hot and humid as midday approached on that spring day in South Florida. There was no shade, and the temperature on the roof was scorching hot. The ground level was no bargain.*

*Our work group took a break for lunch, when the property owner brought us a couple pepperoni pizzas before noon. By then we'd been laboring for over four hours. The crew was ravenous as we chowed down, leaving no crust behind. I was aware that my co-workers had each a couple of beers as well, not something that seemed smart to me. A Diet Coke was more to my liking.*

*The afternoon was dedicated to carrying, lifting, and installing the new materials. There was no power lift, so I got to make endless trips up an extension ladder carrying rolls of tar paper, roofing shingles, and heavy-duty staples and nails for the guns being used to secure the new roof. This process brought with it new hazards. I could slip off the ladder. A work buddy could fall on top of me while I was handing him a load. If he didn't get a firm grip on a stack of shingles being passed his way, they could cause us both to careen onto a concrete patio. I had not anticipated the need to be wary of nail gun projectiles being shot in a reckless manner by a worker who was in a big hurry.*

*The end of the workday came later than expected. We finished the job around 6 p.m. I was beat when the crew chief paid me in cash. I earned an extra ten bucks for my long day in the sun. I recall he was very complimentary when announcing that my services were wanted for another job the next weekend. I responded with, "No thanks. I'd only blame myself if I returned and got hurt. God bless you guys." That was the end of my career as a roofer, the shortest job I ever held.*

## Why Roofing Is So Dangerous

According to the National Institute of Occupational Safety & Health (NIOSH), the leading cause of fatal accidents in roofers is falls. Falls from roofs, ladders, and scaffolding are common. Proper attention to worker safety can prevent many serious accidents.[1] Slip and fall accidents can also result in fractures, connective tissue lesions, damage to internal organs, and head trauma. Serious roofing injuries also commonly occur due to electrocution, burns, and heat exhaustion.

## The Case of Jose Sanchez: Multiple Opinions Causing Confusion

He had been working as a roofer for a decade when Jose Sanchez fell off a roof. He landed on his buttocks, and while sore, he was glad he had not broken any bones that he knew of. As the crew chief, Jose resumed work on that job only to quit after a couple more hours. It was obvious that he was really hurting. The day after his fall, the injured roofer was seen at Urgent Care of Northern California. A basic work-up led to a decision to initiate a workers' comp claim and make a referral to a respected orthopedist.

"Good day, Jose, I'm Dr. Williams. I've got good news and bad news," the injured roofer recalled. That fall on his butt had done significant damage to the area of Jose's lumbosacral spine.

Imaging studies had been ordered, and the first of many opioid narcotic prescriptions to come was waiting for the worker at Walgreen's. The good news was that this injury to his low back could have been much worse.

Weeks away from work dragged into months. Injections at two levels of Jose's lumbar spine had not reduced the worker's pain. Electrodiagnostic studies demonstrated nerve root impingement. Jose reluctantly agreed to undergo surgery that was limited to one level of his spine. It had to get better, but it didn't. One year into a new existence of being labeled an injured worker, Jose found himself struggling with his emotions, self-image, and feelings of hopelessness.

His state disability benefits had run out. Jose hired an attorney after his surgeon advised him to get representation. That didn't make it smooth sailing. In his mid-forties, Jose applied for Social Security Disability benefits. He had been out of the workforce for a dozen years when he was told he'd be meeting with a psychiatrist to assess his state of mind. "I'm not loco. I hurt all the time, " he protested. And so, this simple hard-working man became the subject of clinicians dissecting the corpse of his now-defunct former self. Physical medicine, internal medicine, vocational rehabilitation, and psychiatric experts weighed in as to how disabled the roofer was as the result of his acute work-related injury and all that followed from that life-changing event.

It was a group of blind men touching different parts of the elephant. Was there overlap with what other experts had described? Was there a basis to attribute responsibility to other causes aside from the fall from the roof? If so, how much? Let us parse this and consider that. Jose came to give up any real hope for justice. Yet it was a decision at an appeals level that was in his favor. That decision found it was speculative that nonindustrial factors, whether physical or mental, had brought forth his inability to compete in the labor force.

No one can take joy in Jose being removed from gainful employment, not even halfway through his life expectancy, yet under America's system of justice, he would not be blamed. There was a semblance of vindication for the victim of a severe industrial injury not being cast out for just doing his job. In practical terms, the appeals court decision would make a difference in the benefits Jose and his family would receive.

> *This roofer's saga reminds me of my great-grandfather, who died building the Lincoln Park Lagoon on Chicago's Northside. As "legal aliens," the Iacobuccis were deported as there were no other members of that Italian laborer's family who were employable. Life ain't fair. My family is tough. They came back to the States. With time, maybe there has been some improvement when incurring serious injuries at work in America. However, as seen in cases of Jose Sanchez and my great-grandfather, the personal price to the injured worker can be exceedingly high.*

## The Case of Armando Ramirez: The Painful Truth About Burn Injuries

In his homeland of Mexico, Armando Ramirez attended a public school only through the fifth grade. He then went to work at a fast-food restaurant. He initially worked in a similar job after coming to California at age twenty. He subsequently worked for a janitorial service for a few years. When he had the opportunity to take a union roofing job, Armando was glad to have employment with benefits. One downside to working as a roofer is the rainy season that lasts much of the winter in northern California. This worker usually got some temp work or collected unemployment benefits when the roofing business was slow.

After five years working as a union roofer, Armando took a new job with North Bay Roofing. This company was involved in residential and commercial projects. He had been with that employer for only a few months when he was working on replacing a roof with a team of co-workers and tragedy struck. Armando tripped while carrying a bucket of hot tar. The thick, steamy liquid poured into the glove of his right hand. As he cried out in pain, co-workers helped remove the glove and immerse his affected dominant hand into cool water. It took some time for the ambulance to arrive. On the way to a general hospital that had a burn unit, the roofer was given morphine for his pain.

Initial surgery involved debriding of burned skin, followed by skin grafting using a donor site from Armando's right thigh. Over the next two years, he underwent additional surgery to address scars and contractures of ligaments and tendons. He relied upon opiate painkillers along with medication to combat anxiety, depression, disturbed sleep, and intrusive memories of his work-related accident. A course of short-term psychotherapy helped this roofer take steps to reduce his reliance on medication. He was weaned off the opiate with his attending 12-step meetings for months.

It became clear that the nerve damage to Armando's hand was so extensive that impairments for gripping, grasping, and finger movements would be permanent. The sight of his right hand was also a source of embarrassment for Armando. Orthopedic, neurologic, and plastic surgery experts agreed that this man could not return to any job that required the use of two arms and hands. He was done as a roofer. His prospects for retraining given his limited education were dismal.

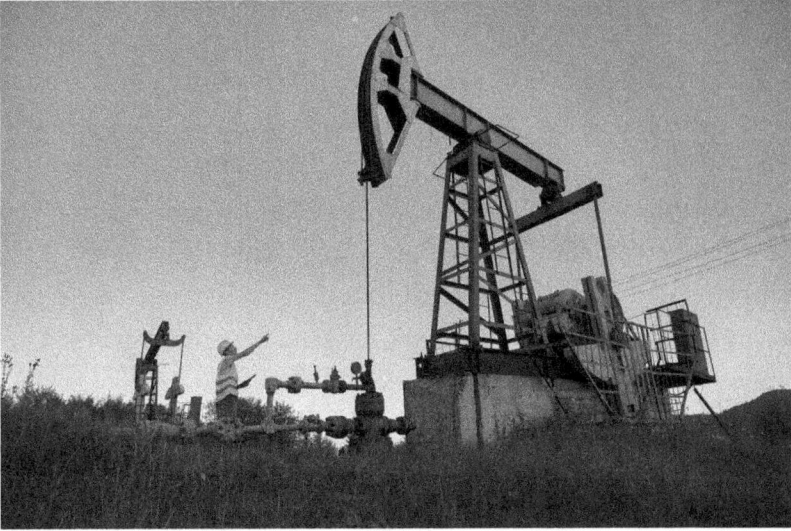

# 23 Derrick Operators: A Crush in Time

## The Dangers of Big Things, High Up

**D**errick and crane operators use massive machinery to move big, heavy loads. These operators work in an elevated enclosure; using camera imagery; joystick technology; computer enhancement; and strong magnets, drills, and scoops to dig, lift, move, and construct large-scale objects as project goals. This is not a profession for someone with a fear of heights. Weather contributes to dangerous conditions.

Make no mistake, this is a multitasking job that can involve extremely heavy loads. To move loads as dense as locomotive engines, one is dealing with massive machinery. It's not for everyone. There are numerous ways that derrick operators are injured. If those heavy loads are destabilized, it can spell disaster. Operators are vulnerable when repositioning large objects.[1]

Operators of derricks and cranes can be seriously injured or die due to malfunctioning equipment given the massive factors of weight, height, electricity, and the maintenance of enormous machinery. Major hazards for crane operators include an excessive load, falling materials, and insufficient inspection and maintenance of equipment.[2] The tale that follows involves a construction site accident brought about by an unstable, heavy load that fell to ground level, bringing with it the operator box and its occupant. The vast majority of crane accidents are the result of the crane's load capacity being exceeded. The case of James Canfield highlights the hazards of excessive load and falling materials. Perhaps insufficient inspection and maintenance were also factors.

## The Terrifying Case of James Canfield: A Serious Head Injury

When the load attached to a crane James Canfield was operating careened to the pavement, it pulled the crane's structure with it. James regained consciousness on the ground level of the construction site where he had been working for several weeks. Workers wearing hard hats pulled him free of the operator's box that had towered several stories above where the jumble of steel and cabling now rested. He was dazed and disoriented, had a headache, his ears were ringing, and he could not maintain his balance when standing.

James had recently turned sixty. He had been operating cranes at construction sites and at manufacturing plants for three decades when he survived that crash. He was taken to San

Francisco General Hospital, a trauma center. There, his multiple contusions were recognized along with a concussion or mild traumatic brain injury (TBI). An MRI brain scan revealed a subdural hematoma in the right frontal lobe of his brain.

After two weeks, James was discharged with outpatient follow-up having been arranged. This included a program of rehabilitation that brought about improvement in his abilities to stand up, walk, and keep his balance.

I initially met with James about eighteen months after his accident. "I feel like a baby," the operator slowly stated during that first interview. He had been fitted with bilateral hearing aids. The anticonvulsant gabapentin had been prescribed to help with his post-traumatic headaches and chronic pain related to numerous sprains and lumbar disc pathology. He also came across as depressed and anxious. As his evaluating psychiatrist, I recommended that James be offered a trial of a first-line antidepressant to help stabilize his emotions, improve his sleep, and address his very real pain.

Another couple of years went by before I re-evaluated James. He had completed a course of physical therapy overseen by a specialist trained in physical medicine and rehabilitation. He was wearing a San Francisco Giants baseball cap and a smile when we shook hands. The operator moved about in a deliberate manner, yet he got by without using a cane or walker. Through muscle strengthening exercises and perseverance, James had managed to return to construction worksites. In fact, he was part of a team building the new baseball park at China Basin.

The good news was that James had weaned himself off the anticonvulsant. He had received a new, permanent set of hearing aids. He reported that the use of fluoxetine, an antidepressant, had helped with troubled sleep and emotional volatility. James still had periodic nightmares. He was grateful for the progress he had made since coming close to death, but he still struggled with his attention, concentration, and memory. Those persistent cognitive problems had been discussed with a psychologist. Like his headaches, James came to accept that he would continue to feel sad at times and that his thinking wasn't as sharp as it had been before his TBI.

In his mid-sixties, James had a plan to retire from his long career. He was teaching younger operators to take over in upcoming months. His union and his employer had arranged for a retirement event at the ballpark after it opened. This injured worker would receive a settlement related to his workers' compensation claims. More importantly, he had regained a sense of pride in himself. The accident had left this man with some limitations, but he had not been beaten. He left my office with these words, "Let's go, Giants!"

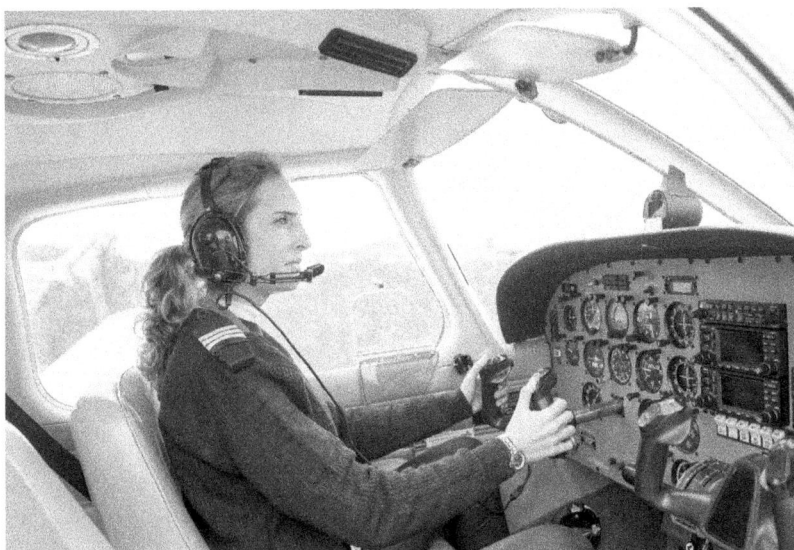

# 24 Pilots: When Aircraft Go Down

## How Hazardous Is Flying Small Aircraft?

Some say the difference in safety measures in the airline industry versus the healthcare industry is enormous. Operator error happens far more often in the E.R. or the O.R. than in the cockpit. When your doctor makes a mistake, he has a second martini when at home. When a pilot makes a mistake, he dies too. Think about it. Physicians have a lot to learn from the professionals who fly planes. It's called zero tolerance for errors. Check, check, and double-check.

According to the Federal Aviation Administration (FAA), the ten most frequent pilot-related factors involved in aviation accidents are inadequate preflight preparation, failure to maintain flying speed, failure to maintain direction control, improper level-off, failure to avoid objects, mismanagement of fuel, poor in-flight decisions, misjudgment of distance/speed, selecting unsuitable terrain, and improper operation of flight controls.[1]

The duties of an aircraft pilot are numerous. Attention to detail is a must, or bad things can happen. Because of their training and safety standards, pilots have a good record for operations errors. Like Boy Scouts, pilots have a plan and follow the plan. No one wants a pilot who is in a hurry. No one wants a pilot who seeks out risk.

## The Tale of Ben Returns

I first told Ben's tale in *Wounded Workers*.[2] The terror of errors in small aircraft can be exemplified by returning to the story of that battalion chief. While determining how much equipment and personnel would be required to fight a massive wildfire, he crashed in a helicopter. Ben was a highly experienced and well-trained professional with a degree in forestry from Cal Berkeley who went airborne with a young pilot who misrepresented his experience and disregarded directives. The young man's arrogance nearly caused Ben's death.

As a result of pilot error, the helicopter that Ben was in hit the treetops and crashed. He was trapped in the wreckage, bleeding out from his wounds, and covered in aviation fuel during a massive wildfire. The pilot and the spotter were thrown free. Ben assessed the situation and decided he was going to die, one way or the other. He prayed that he would bleed to death before the fire ignited the fuel. A group of firefighters dropped their personal safety equipment and rescued Ben.

Medevaced to a trauma center, the battalion chief underwent blood transfusions and multiple surgeries. A long recovery followed. Ben had to learn to walk again. His tale is one of redemption. Never a violent man, Ben learned that the pilot should have dumped or burned off fuel. The copter crashed unnecessarily. Because of his injuries, Ben was prescribed narcotic analgesics. Unfortunately, he became habituated to the painkillers, while mired in anger toward the negligent pilot. He was confronted by his wife. He took her pleas seriously, weaned himself off the narcotics, and forgave the pilot. These were not easy tasks.

Ben's career could have ended with the crash. Instead, he went on to become a member of the Cal Fire Academy, training younger firefighters. In his last position as deputy chief, he oversaw employee assistance, stress management, and peer support services for California firefighters. Some may ask why Ben stayed productive and remained a source of support to colleagues. It's simple. He was raised right. Ben was presented with the Courage Award by the California Society of Industrial Medicine and Surgery in recognition of his resilience and hardiness when continuing his career rather than retiring.

The focus of this chapter is the dangers of being a pilot. Pilot errors are often serious, if not fatal for the pilot. In this case, the pilot caused tragedy for co-workers. Flying aircraft is not for sissies, and mistakes are best minimized.

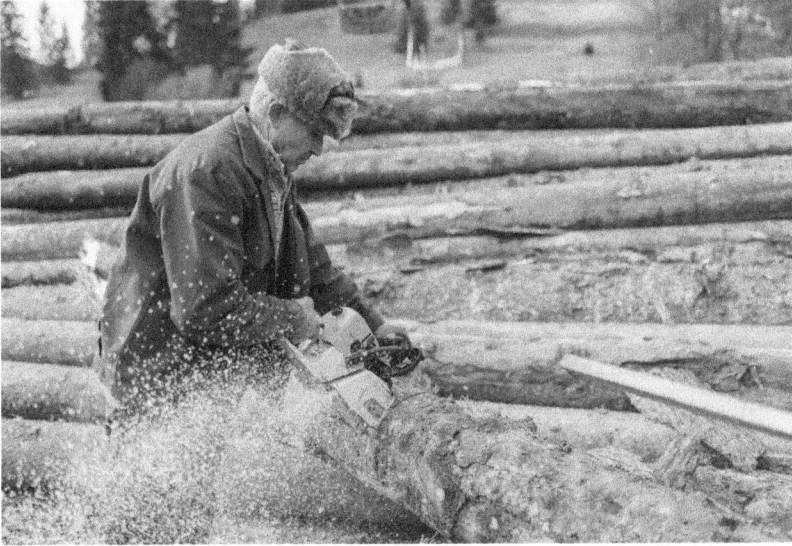

# 25 Logging: America's Most Dangerous Job

## Logging Has High Rates of Fatal and Non-Fatal Injuries

Air in northern California is clean as you approach the border with Oregon. The sounds of chainsaws fill the air. The California redwood and the Douglas fir are majestic to behold and highly prized for their value to the building industry. Loggers have been working these hillsides for generations. The forest workers of the 21$^{st}$ century have roots going back to their great-grandfathers who never held a power tool. Work was dangerous then and remains dangerous now. Treacherous hillsides, enormous careening objects, heavy machinery, and changing conditions all contribute to accidents.

Over a ten-year period, the logging industry had 23 times the fatality rate for all U.S. workers (164 versus 7 deaths per 100,000 workers/FTEs). Due to methods for collecting and reporting data, it is believed the lethal nature of logging is even higher. Logging injuries include those suffered by workers with logging jobs (e.g., fellers, limbers, buckers, and choker setters), truck drivers, laborers, and machine operators.[1] Logging also has the highest total injury rate of more than 14,000 per 100,000 workers versus approximately 8,000 per annum for all private sector jobs.[2] There are many ways to get seriously injured as a logger or forester.[3]

More recent data, from the Bureau of Labor Statistics, continues to find logging to be dangerous when considering fatal injuries and total number of injuries. Logging is grouped with farming and fishing occupations. In 2021, that category had 20.0 fatalities per 100,000 FTE workers. The average across all occupations was 3.6. In 2022, farming, fishing, and logging again had the highest fatality rate at 23.5 deaths per 100,000 workers, with 3.7 being the average across all occupations.[4] *The New York Times* has reported logging to be the most dangerous occupation in the U.S. The industry has declined due to foreign competition from Brazil and Canada as well as from legal disputes with conservationists over old-growth forests.[5]

## The Case of Dale Richards: Big Trees and Powerful Machinery

Dale Richards grew up in Redding, California, where he was one of six kids who were raised in a working-class family. His father worked as a truck mechanic and handyman when the economy was good. Dale was assigned to special education classes and was made fun of by some of his peers. He liked the outdoors and enjoyed playing baseball but never tried out for competitive sports as a teen. He had little experience dating. After finishing high school, Dale had a series of entry level jobs as a construction laborer, a tire junkie, a welder, and a loading dock worker. As a young adult, he incurred a mild traumatic brain injury as the result of a multi-vehicle accident that led to him being out of the workforce for several months. Then he got a job with Jim's Tree Service based in Arcata. He took to the work as he enjoyed spending time in the lush forests of Humboldt County.

Dale worked for several logging companies over a period of a half dozen years. He had a reputation for getting the job done. He could fell trees with a chainsaw, set chokers, and operate heavy equipment such as specially equipped tractors. He had been with his current, and last, employer for only a month when he became a logging industry statistic.

Dale was working as a member of a small crew. He was on the ground while his co-worker was operating a tractor equipped with a blade that was used to push against the base of large fir trees. The first few trees came down as expected. The last one began to topple unexpectedly toward Dale. Unable to avert being crushed by outrunning the falling behemoth, the logger leapt toward the blade of the tractor, to dive under it. The tractor operator panicked and lowered the blade, which came to rest on Dale's right leg. Dale was bleeding from the area of a compound fracture of his crushed limb. The crew extracted their injured comrade. There was no time to waste cleaning off soil from the forest floor.

The initial hospitalization involved debriding the leg wound, performing vascular surgery to address hemorrhaging from the femoral artery, the transfusion of multiple units of blood, and an above-the-knee amputation. Dale survived, yet he would never work as a logger again. Additional surgeries were required to stabilize the stump site where he would be fitted with a prosthesis. After several fittings at the University of California, San Francisco Medical Center, an acceptable artificial limb was found that allowed Dale some semblance of mobility without finding himself limited by pain.

It was pain that had led to his taking a fair number and total amount of narcotics. His doctors advised that Dale consult with a psychologist back home. He underwent some psychological testing that confirmed he was struggling with symptoms of depression, anxiety, and embarrassment over his prosthetic limb. His psychologist helped her patient to venture out in public while wearing his bionic leg. With time, he started wearing shorts as he came to accept his new appearance. A psychiatrist assisted in reducing Dale's use of pain and sleep medication with a sedating antidepressant helping to limit potentially addictive pharmaceuticals. None of these developments came about easily.

Dale's acute injuries stabilized, and six years post-injury, his workers' compensation case was settled. Dale, now a former logger, ended up receiving Social Security benefits. He had begun taking courses at the local junior college though he was uncertain what type of alternative work he might ever be able to take on. He had been evaluated in our offices for the psychiatric issues that left him with lingering moodiness characterized by feelings of frustration and resentment. We determined his persistent emotional distress was the result of a compensable consequence psychiatric injury related to his primary physical injuries of an orthopedic, vascular, and medical nature.

The case of Dale Richards shows how tenuous our existence can be. Do you take for granted your ability to walk about, as the logger had before he lost his leg? We use denial as a means of coping with the possibility that an event related to our job duties can leave us both less functional and less independent. There was no magical outcome in Dale's situation, brought about by a single bad day on the job.

> *For Dale Richards and many other wounded workers portrayed in this compendium of dangerous jobs, the outcome is a career-ending injury. "All the King's horses and all the King's men couldn't put Humpty Dumpty back together again." This adage is not intended to demean these seriously injured workers. Instead, it is meant as a recognition that most working people are in denial about how a single accident or a series of traumas can permanently change one's existence.*
>
> *We all know we are mortal, yet we would rather not even imagine having to confront life-changing disability, or worse, just showing up at the worksite. Social Security is a social welfare system that provides more than expected retirement benefits. For those employees who cannot be put back together again, federal, state, and private disability programs can prevent poverty from adding further to an already troubling tale.*

## The Case of Grant Graham: Forced to Adapt

As a young man in his mid-twenties, Grant Graham was challenged by the injury he incurred as a logger in northern California. He grew up in Humboldt County where his father was the manager of a lumber mill while his mother was a member of a commercial fishing crew. Grant really didn't apply himself throughout high school, yet he graduated. He went to work in the logging industry because there were plenty of jobs available, though they tended to be seasonal due to a long rainy season.

Grant has memories as a four- or five-year old accompanying his father into the lush woods where loggers could choose enormous specimens to harvest. By the time he was logging in his late teens, Grant was familiar with chain saws, delimbers, chippers, mulchers, and several special tools used by forestry workers. While he remained in the area where he grew up, Grant tended to stay with an employer for a year or two before moving on. He had been with Ashland Logging since the spring. Months later, toward the end of the logging season in October, he got hurt.

While clearing a logging path for his crew, Grant was selectively cutting down trees. A strong breeze came up, causing the tree he was cutting down to fall prematurely. Grant looked for a clear path to take. Turning his head, he was struck by falling debris from nearby trees. He experienced intense pain around his left eye and could feel with his gloved hand that his eyeball was protruding out of its socket.

Members of his crew acted quickly in taking Grant to a local hospital. The initial surgery addressed the facial lacerations but could not save the damaged eye.

By the time I met with Grant, he had undergone four facial surgeries and had been fitted with a prosthetic eye. It had been a year and a half since he last worked in the woods. He had stopped using prescription medication for his pain. With the support of a counselor, he had given up using an eye patch while being careful that his prosthetic eye was positioned properly. He admitted to having some sensitivity about his appearance when out in public. That was also a topic addressed in his every-other-week sessions with that same counselor.

Losing vision in one eye results in a loss of depth perception. That alone made it impossible for Grant to resume work as a logger. While he could adapt to an extent, he needed to be more deliberate when moving about to avoid bumping into things. Counseling had led him back to school with the intention of completing courses for an associate's degree. That achievement would allow him to enroll at a state university. His goal was to obtain a bachelor's degree in resource management. Grant was proud of making the dean's list at the community college. His parents were supportive and helping financially.

The psychological test results were consistent with an admixture of mild depression and anxiety. Grant admitted to making use of medicinal marijuana, which helped with anxiety about his appearance. Otherwise, he seemed to have channeled his frustration and uncertainty into a plan for a future where he expected to be productive and independent. I recommended that Grant continue in counseling while the insurer would cover the costs of college course work. This amounted to a vocational rehabilitation plan that would result in a return of a young adult to the workforce, who would otherwise be displaced and disabled.

*Count your blessings rather than focus on how life could be better. Don't live in fear of injury and insult. However, try to appreciate that the health you have is not guaranteed. Eat right, exercise, and work at maintaining your body, mind, and soul's good functioning. Be your own best advocate by recognizing potential hazards. If you become a wounded worker, take seriously the consequences that follow. Assemble a team of professionals you trust. Nothing is more important than fighting for your employment rights and your optimal health.*

# Postscript

**Imagine the following tale. Maria had been our** neighbor's housekeeper after they settled in New Mexico two decades ago. She preferred to be paid in cash. She and her husband of twenty-some years operated under the radar. They came to the U.S. on work visas. To renew their documentation, they were expected to return to El Salvador for a time. However, the couple had married, and Maria gave birth to a baby boy, Tony, who was an American citizen. As a couple, Tony's parents did not want to risk being separated from him. They didn't renew their visas, yet they continued to work, pay taxes, and stay out of trouble. Or so they thought. Carlos, the housekeeper's mate, was a skilled construction worker. Ten years after the birth of their son, the couple welcomed a baby girl into their family. The kids were U.S. citizens as provided by law per the 14th Amendment to our country's Constitution.

Things got complicated after Carlos injured his nondominant, left hand when a co-worker using an electric drill accidentally pierced that appendage. The radial nerve was severed. The employer apparently didn't carry workers' comp insurance for Carlos, adding further complexity to a disabling injury. This injured worker didn't feel safe getting treated for his injury after our President was making good on his campaign promise to round up and deport illegal immigrants. This family of four now lived in terror of being split up. Their son had begun college on a scholarship that might be in jeopardy of disappearing. The younger daughter, in grammar school, could be forced to live apart from her parents, should they be deported.

This story has been repeated across America. It is not the tale of violent criminals being held responsible for their bad deeds, but of decent folks looking for a better life in the dreamland that became a nightmare. As the son of an immigrant who became an American, I had heard my ma's story of her grandfather dying from an industrial accident in Chicago. His widow and children were sent back to Italy when there was no longer a family member who could do heavy labor. Life isn't always fair. A generation later, my mother's family returned to stay. Immigrants can be tough and determined.

Immigrants often do the jobs that third-generation Americans don't find attractive. They pick the crops, clean our houses, collect the garbage, and take on a myriad of tasks that don't pay well while being fraught with the potential for serious injury. Once regarded as the Land of Opportunity, America is gaining a different reputation for greed and indifference. "Give us your tired, your poor, your huddled masses yearning to breathe free." Was this beacon of liberty no longer operative? Time would tell.

Several of the tales in *America's Most Dangerous Jobs* involve recent immigrants or their immediate descendants. They work as roofers, loggers, maintenance workers, and cooks. I worked one day as a roofer before I quit that endeavor due to its obvious hazards. How many of us would aspire to pick up trash or clean toilets for a living? Those who risk their health for showing up at the worksite deserve to have their stories told.

In *Wounded Workers*, the tales of employees injured physically and psychologically were begun as a means of honoring the sacrifice made by those who might otherwise be forgotten. My hope is that, through storytelling, we become more sensitive to those around us who provide goods and services that we depend on. None of the workers portrayed wanted to end their careers as a result of impairment, disability or worse. These sagas may remind us that, "There, but for the grace of God, go I."

# Notes

*All web links were accessed in March 2025.*

## Introduction

1.  "Civilian Occupations with High Fatal Work Injury Rates," U.S. Bureau of Labor Statistics, *bls.gov* : 2024 (https://www.bls.gov/charts/census-of-fatal-occupational-injuries/civilian-occupations-with-high-fatal-work-injury-rates.htm).

2.  Adrian Mak, "Top 25 Most Dangerous Jobs in the United States," *Advisor Smith* : September 30, 2021 (https://advisorsmith.com/data/most-dangerous-jobs/).

3.  Benita Mehta, "The Top 25 Most Dangerous Jobs in the United States," *Industrial Safety & Hygeine News* : November 5, 2020

(https://www.ishn.com/articles/112748-top-25-most-dangerous-jobs-in-the-united-states).

4. "The 10 Most Dangerous Jobs in America," *CNBC* : December 27, 2019 (https://www.cnbc.com/2019/12/27/the-10-most-dangerous-jobs-in-america-according-to-bls-data.html).

5. "Census of Fatal Occupational Injuries for 2022," U.S. Bureau of Labor Statistics, *bls.gov* : December 2023 (https://www.bls.gov/iif/fatal-injuries-tables/fatal-occupational-injuries-table-a-7-2023.htm).

## 1: Construction Workers

1. "Why is working in construction so dangerous?" *LetsBuild* : October 18, 2023 (https://www.letsbuild.com/blog/working-construction-dangerous).

2. Jill Fleming, "The Biggest Danger in Construction Work Is Poor Mental Health," *EHS Today* : August 3, 2021 (https://www.ehstoday.com/construction/article/21171410/the-biggest-danger-in-construction-work-is-poor-mental-heath).

## 2: Mining Machine Operators

1. "Mining in the United States," *The Diggings* : undated (https://thediggings.com/usa).

2. "U.S. Mining Industry," *American Mine Services* : undated (https://americanmineservices.com/us-mining-industry).

## 3: Maintenance Workers

1. Khaled Ismail, "Maintaining Your Safety for Maintenance Workers," *HSSE World* : December 10, 2021 (https://hsseworld.com/maintaining-your-safety-for-maintenance-workers/).

## 4: Police Officers

1. "Officer Safety," National Institute of Justice, *nij.ojp.gov* : undated (https://nij.ojp.gov/topics/law-enforcement/officer-safety).

## 5: Grounds Maintenance Workers

1. Stephen S. Pegula, "Occupational Injuries among Groundskeepers, 1992–2002," U.S. Bureau of Labor Statistics, *bls.gov* : December 20, 2005 (https://www.bls.gov/opub/mlr/cwc/occupational-injuries-among-groundskeepers-1992-2002.pdf).

## 6: Heavy Equipment Mechanics

1. Devin Partida, "5 Dangers of Working Around Heavy Equipment and How to Stay Safe," Occupational Health and Safety, *ohsonline.com* : August 12, 2021 (https://ohsonline.com/Articles/2021/08/12/5-Dangers-of-Working-Around-Heavy-Equipment-and-How-to-Stay-Safe.aspx).

## 7: Supervisors of Mechanics

1. "Mechanical Maintenance Supervisor Skills for Your Resume and Career," *Zippia* : February 16, 2024 (https://www.zippia.com/mechanical-maintenance-supervisor-jobs/skills/).

2. Pamela Reynolds, "Preventing and Managing Team Conflict," *Harvard Division of Continuing Education* : October 31, 2022 (https://professional.dce.harvard.edu/blog/preventing-and-managing-team-conflict/).

## 8: Small-Engine Mechanics

1. "Small Engine Mechanics," U.S. Bureau of Labor Statistics, *bls.gov* : August 29, 2024 (https://www.bls.gov/ooh/installation-maintenance-and-repair/small-engine-mechanics.htm).

2. "Workplace Carbon Monoxide Hazards," National Institute for Occupational Safety and Health, *cdc.gov* : September 30, 2024 (https://www.cdc.gov/niosh/carbon-monoxide/about/).

## 9: Cement Masons

1. "Masonry Workers," U.S. Bureau of Labor Statistics, *bls.gov* : August 29, 2024 (https://www.bls.gov/ooh/construction-and-

extraction/brickmasons-blockmasons-and-stonemasons.htm).

## 10: Highway Maintenance Workers

1. "Highway Work Zone Safety," National Institute for Occupational Safety and Health, *cdc.gov* : November 6, 2024 (https://www.cdc.gov/niosh/motor-vehicle/highway/).

## 11: Landscaping Supervisors

1. "Landscape and Horticultural Services: Hazards and Solutions," Occupational Safety and Health Administration, *osha.gov* : undated (https://www.osha.gov/landscaping/hazards).

## 12: Construction Helpers

1. Nichole Helmick and Jeremy Petosa. "Workplace Injuries and Job Requirements for Construction Workers," U.S. Bureau of Labor Statistics, *bls.gov* : November 2022 (https://www.bls.gov/spotlight/2022/workplace-injuries-and-job-requirements-for-construction-laborers/).

2. Scott Schneider. "Looking into a New Year of Construction Laborer Injury Data," Laborers' Health and Safety Fund of North America : January 1, 2021 (https://lhsfna.org/looking-into-a-new-year-of-construction-laborer-injury-data/).

3. Marcela Valdes, Churchill Ndonwie, Danielle Ivory, and Steve Eder. "Fatal Accidents for Immigrants in U.S. Factories," *New York Times* : December 22, 2024, p. 1 (https://www.nytimes.com/2024/12/21/us/immigration-undocumented-workers-jobs.html).

## 13: Crane Operators

1. Dan Drummond. "Common Crane Safety Hazards: 5 Top Safety Concerns When Operating a Crane," General Construction Crane Service, *generalcranect.com* (https://generalcranect.com/crane-safety-hazards/) : September 30, 2020 and Leon Altamonte, "A

Comprehensive Guide to Crane Safety," Safety Culture : December 13, 2023 (https://safetyculture.com/topics/crane-safety).

2. Robert Larsen, *Wounded Workers: Tales from a Working Man's Shrink* (Santa Fe: Working Man's Press, 2021).

## 14: Crossing Guards

1. David Wylie, "4 Safety Tips for Crossing Guards," TASB Risk Fund, *tasbrmf.org* : July 28, 2022 (https://www.tasbrmf.org/resources/insights/4-safety-tips-for-crossing-guards).

## 15: Farm Workers

1. "Rural Agricultural Health and Safety," Rural Health Information Hub, *ruralhealthinfo.org* (https://www.ruralhealthinfo.org/topics/agricultural-health-and-safety).

## 16: Power Line Workers

1. Yaakov Daskal, Alexander Beicker, Mickey Dudkiewicz, and Boris Kessel, "High Voltage Electric Injury: Mechanism of Injury, Clinical Features and Initial Evaluation," National Library of Medicine, *nlm.nih.gov* : January 2019 (https://pubmed.ncbi.nlm.nih.gov/30663297/).

2. Brian J. Daley, "Electrical Injuries," *Medscape* : November 6, 2024 (https://emedicine.medscape.com/article/433682).

## 17: Firefighters

1. Paul A. Demers, David M. DeMarini, Kenneth W. Fent, Deborah C. Glass, Johnni Hansen, Olorunfemi Adetona, et al. "Carcinogenicity of Occupational Exposure as a Firefighter," *Lancet Oncology*, 23:8, August 2022; published online: June 30, 2022 (https://doi.org/10.1016/S1470-2045(22)00390-4).

2. Dierdre Lockwood, "Preventing long-term health risks for firefighters," *Environmental & Occupational Health Sciences* : January 23, 2023 (https://deohs.washington.edu/hsm-blog/preventing-long-

term-health-risks-firefighters).

## 18: Farmers and Ranchers

1. R. J. Fetsch, "Farming, Ranching: Health Hazard or Opportunity?" Colorado State University Extension, *colostate. edu* : June 2011 (https://extension.colostate.edu/docs/pubs/ consumer/10201.pdf).

2. Nicholas Bogel-Burroughs, "'Pretty Sickening': Texas Ranchers Face Sickening Losses," *New York Times* : March. 2, 2024 (https://www.nytimes.com/2024/03/02/us/texas-fires-rancher. html).

## 19: Delivery Drivers

1. "Common Delivery Driver Accidents and Injuries, National Accident Helpline" (https://www.national-accident-helpline.co.uk/ news/post/common-delivery-driver-accidents-injuries).

2. Robert Larsen, *Wounded Workers: Tales from a Working Man's Shrink* (Santa Fe: Working Man's Press, 2021).

## 20: Ironworkers

1. Les Christie. "America's Most Dangerous Jobs: Ironworkers," *CNN Business* : August 22, 2013 (https://money.cnn.com/gallery/pf/ jobs/2013/08/22/dangerous-jobs/5.html).

## 21: Refuse and Recyclable Collectors

1. Emily Atkins, "Waste worker fatalities climbed in 2022," *Waste & Recycling* : March 8, 2023 (https://wasterecyclingmag.ca/ health-and-safety/worker-fatalities-climbed-in-2022/1003288365/).

2. "Industries at a Glance: Waste Management and Remediation Services: NAICS 562," U.S. Bureau of Labor Statistics, *bls.gov* : March 28, 2025 (https://www.bls.gov/iag/tgs/iag562.htm).

## 22: Roofing

1. "Prevent Construction Falls from Roofs, Ladders, and Scaffolds," National Institute for Occupational Safety and Health, *cdc.gov*, Pub. No. 2019–128 : November 15, 2019 (https://www.cdc.gov/niosh/docs/2019-128/).

## 23: Derrick Operators

1. "Crane, Derrick and Hoist Safety," Occupational Safety and Health Administration, *osha.gov* : undated (https://www.osha.gov/cranes-derricks/hazards).

2. Michele Kienle. "Top 3 Major Crane Hazards and How to Avoid Them." American Crane & Equipment Corp. : December 19, 2019 (https:// https://www.americancrane.com/top-3-major-crane-hazards-and-how-to-avoid-them/).

## 24: Pilots

1. "Aeronautical Information Publication: ENR 5.7, Potential Flight Hazards," Federal Aviation Administration : undated (https://www.faa.gov/air_traffic/publications/atpubs/aip_html/part2_enr_section_5.7.html).

2. Robert Larsen, *Wounded Workers: Tales from a Working Man's Shrink* (Santa Fe: Working Man's Press, 2021).

## 25: Logging

1. "Preventing Injuries and Deaths of Loggers," National Institute for Occupational Safety and Health, *cdc.gov*, Pub. No. 95–101 (https://www.cdc.gov/niosh/docs/95-101/).

2. *Ibid.*, citing NIOSH [1993a]. "National traumatic occupational fatalities (NTOF) surveillance system." National Institute for Occupational Safety and Health, *cdc.gov*, unpublished database.

3. *Ibid.*, citing NIOSH [1993b], "Fatal Injuries to Workers in the United States, 1980–1989: A Decade of Surveillance —

179

National and State Profiles," National Institute for Occupational Safety and Health, *cdc.gov*, Pub. No. 93-108S (https://www.cdc.gov/niosh/docs/93-108s/default.html); and BLS [1994], "Survey of Occupational Injuries and Illnesses, 1992," U.S. Bureau of Labor Statistics, *bls.gov*, Pub. No. 94–3 : May 1994 (updated annually at: https://www.bls.gov/news.release/cfoi.nr0.htm ; archived at: https://babel.hathitrust.org/cgi/pt?id=mdp.39015032125679&seq=1).

4. *Ibid.,* citing BLS [2023,] "National Census of Fatal Occupational Injuries, 2022," U.S. Bureau of Labor Statistics, *bls.gov*, Pub. No. 94–3 : Dec. 2023 (updated annually at: https://www.bls.gov/news.release/cfoi.nr0.htm ; archived at: https://web.archive.org/web/20231228215118/https://www.bls.gov/news.release/cfoi.nr0.htm).

5. Kurtis Lee and Kristina Barker, "Inside the Deadliest Job in America," *New York Times* : November 22, 2024 (https://www.nytimes.com/2024/11/22/business/economy/logging-oregon-job-danger.html).

# Acknowledgments

My career has been spent as a physician and psychiatrist serving an employee population that has paid a high price for doing their jobs. These tales speak for themselves and hopefully convince those who read them to recognize the sacrifices made.

To my wife, Kim, I owe much for encouraging me throughout my writing projects, now culminating in the publication of *America's Most Dangerous Jobs.* My office manager, Wendy Lemberg, has kept the cases organized and secure, while assisting with gathering information related to this project. Wendy is also the organizational bedrock of my clinical practice from which all these tales emanate. Many of the psychological insights

181

of the book's tales are the product of my long-time psychology associate, Dr. Eric Morgenthaler.

A number of colleagues have reviewed early versions of the manuscript in progress. This includes my long-time fellow physicians Drs. Mike Post and Steve Feinberg, experts in pain management and physical medicine, respectively. Dr. Joel Fay is a psychologist who is the lead clinician at a retreat for first responders whose expertise is relevant to the tales of cops and firefighters portrayed in Chapters 4 and 17. Julius Young is an attorney who has represented injured workers throughout a long career. Julius has cheered me on in getting out this message of sacrifice made by the folks he represents. Anne Hillerman, a friend and best-selling author, has invited you to learn from these tales of employees whose emotional distress is as real as any physical pain.

Jim Wagner provided proofreading of an early draft, as he had done for *Wounded Workers*. My friend and fellow psychiatrist, Dr. David Baron, has penned a personal note that is the foreword to this nonfiction narrative. Exterior design has relied upon the services of Irene and Brianna at Graphic Sky Printing. Kiera Miller selected the interior images and promoted this project through eBlasts and Musings from Working Man's Press.

Finally, the collaboration with my editor, Jordan Jones of Coyote Arts in Albuquerque, has been invaluable. Jordan has edited, designed, and shepherded this writing project to fruition. I am forever grateful that I live in a community where Jordan is a fellow member of the New Mexico Book Association, a great group of professionals who love the art of a well-turned phrase.

With gratitude for making these tales come to life. Enjoy the read, Dr. Bob Larsen

# About the Author

Over a career of four decades, Dr. Bob Larsen has evaluated, treated, and advocated for multitudes of injured workers. Bob Larsen grew up a working-class kid in the Chicago area. He headed west to study cell biology at the University of Colorado. He then engaged in basic science research at the University of Miami, Boston University, and Northwestern University, where he taught microbiology to his fellow medical school classmates. It was early in his medical training that Dr. Bob became enamored of psychiatry through the mentorship of Drs. Hal Visotsky and Francois Alouf.

Following residency training at the University of California, San Francisco (UCSF), a fellowship in health policy at Stanford and UCSF, and graduate studies in healthcare administration at the University of California, Berkeley, Dr. Bob opted to take a hands-on approach to being a psychiatrist serving the needs of injured workers. Workers from all sectors of employment have been referred to his practice as a result of bank robberies, officer-involved shootings, amputation of limbs, and numerous other workplace horrors.

Dr. Bob has been a treating physician, a health policy advocate, an educator, and a forensic psychiatrist. He taught forensic psychiatry as a clinical professor at UCSF. He founded the Center for Occupational Psychiatry in 1985. He is past president of the California Society of Industrial Medicine and Surgery and served as the psychiatric appointee to the Industrial Medical Council of California for the entirety of its thirteen-year existence. His body of professional work is portrayed in *Wounded Workers*. *America's Most Dangerous Jobs* now brings to life the sacrifice made by American workers for just doing their jobs. Those jobs are frequently more dangerous than is commonly known or acknowledged.

Apart from his clinical duties, writing projects, and speaking engagements, Dr. Bob enjoys sharing life with his wife, Kim, in the community of Santa Fe, New Mexico. His avocational interests include photography, travel, blues music, baseball, and creating spray-painted yard art. Those non-clinical pursuits are credited with helping Dr. Bob to "keep on keepin' on."

For more information on Dr. Bob Larsen through his writings, musings, and appearances, visit his website at https://www.workingmansshrink.com.